LITERALLY... UNTIL DEATH

PULLING BACK THE CURTAIN ON CHEMO SIDE-EFFECTS

By
Kim Henderly

Marie —
Thank you for your kindness
and support! Please
help me get this word!
Pump up the Volume &
fight like a Girl!
Be Well
Kim Henderly

2 MOON Press

MARSHALL - MICHIGAN
800PUBLISHING.COM

Literally... Until Death: Pulling Back the Curtain on Chemo Side-Effects

Cover design by Don Semora www.DonSemora.com

Layout by Kait Lamphere

Edited by Sean P. Hobbs and Hannah Moeggenborg

Author photo courtesy of author

ISBN-13: 978-1-938110-81-8

First published in 2012

10 9 8 7 6 5 4 3 2 1

Published by 2 MOON PRESS
123 W. Michigan Ave, Marshall, Michigan 49068
www.800publishing.com

Dedicated to:

Chris Henderly
The love of my life. My Other Half.

And

Hunter Henderly
Because you didn't have to say
what you did, but you did.

I love you both with all my heart and soul.

Edited by:

Sean P. Hobbs

"There is a long black granite wall in Washington DC… The Vietnam Memorial Wall… and not to take anything away from anyone who gave their life in service of this great country… but that wall is about 500 feet long-about a football field and a half- got a good picture of it in your mind? It would take TEN of those walls ONCE A YEAR to list the names of all the people who die in the CANCER WAR"

- Kim Henderly

  Excerpt from the speech given at the Taylor, MI 2011 Relay for Life

Hi

My name is Kim Henderly…

and I am a Cancer Veteran…

CONTENTS

INTRODUCTION

As I sat with my laptop, the keys making that little clicking sound for hours, and hours, I put down all my thoughts about what was happening around me and to me as I started this process. The same question kept coming up in my head as well as in the thoughts of those who I told I was writing this book—*"What is it about?"*

I always had a quick answer to those who asked:

"I have to let people know how all-encompassing this is. How many people are infected, and how incredibly horrific the treatment is. It's like some big secret."

Before I even began this rambling of happenings and thoughts, as I was bombarded early on with a flood of info and a catalogue of medicines. I read. By that, I mean anything I could get my hands on: every book written by a cancer veteran, all the internet blogs, the medical sites, hospital web-pages, and cancer informational pages and brochures.

There is so much information out there. Most of it is dated, one-sided to promote a specific agenda, or just plain incorrect. The books, although I believe written like mine with the best intentions, leave the reader with a false sense of hope and many will promote Vegetarian and Health lifestyles as 'the cure.' These things are incredibly important but they go hand in hand with the medical side of cancer care. THERE IS NO CURE FOR CANCER.

You have to know that what I am expressing in these pages is what I have tried to tell every person I have come in contact with. Most looked at me with a pitying face and tried to humor my ideas but never really comprehending or understanding the viciousness, of what I was saying. A casual conversation will not reveal the true devastation that one's entire life goes through when diagnosed with certain cancers.

According to the major players in the war on cancer, this disease, in all its forms, will affect 1 in 2 women and 1 in 3 men or about 41% of the American population within the next decade. Cancer deaths are second behind heart disease, and about a quarter of those people who are diagnosed with cancer won't make it to the five year survival mark.

Those numbers are always marred in rhetoric and some organization's need for the almighty dollar. Let me be blunt here, they are in plain common sense terms…

In the next ten years…

Just under half of the people in America will get some form of cancer

A quarter of those people will die from cancer.

Do you have five people you are close to in your family? Pick…. two get cancer and one gets to die from that cancer…..

Are you starting to get the idea? Are you scared? You should be.

I knew those numbers going into my diagnosis. I was educated. I could even tell you percentages. Yet I didn't understand them and the enormity of this disease or even how they related to a particular cancer.

The most important thing to understand about cancer is what the treatment of this disease does to you. If the cancer doesn't kill you, the treatment of it will make a *run for your life.*

There was a whole network of people who appeared to me after my diagnosis. Friends, family, strangers—each inflicted with some form of cancer who came forward to offer support and help, yet when I started asking direct questions, they avoided giving direct answers. The medical professionals were even worse. I ran into a standard statement—"everybody's different." I say medical professionals are controlled by the lawyers who run the hospitals and everyday people are embarrassed to talk about the treatment and what it does to you.

Guess what…

I'm not embarrassed.

CHAPTER ONE
THE FAT CHICK

I am not sure when it all started. I do not have that long dragged out story that makes for good reading. You know the one: *I had some sort of mystery illness, and doctor after doctor thought it was all in my head.*

It didn't work that way for me. You see, I am a big girl. Let's be real. I am fat. Not the way you might be picturing…the buffet-eating, –potato-chip-swallowing, soda-pop-guzzling, 400-pound mess. No, I am a 5 foot 10 inches and 248 pounds kind of fat. Now that's a big girl.

I wasn't always that way. I spent the majority of my adult life hovering between 204 and 225. (Yes, fat people know their exact weight. How else can they lie about it?) Quite frankly, if I was a man and just under six feet tall, we wouldn't even be having this talk. However, I am not a man, so it is important.

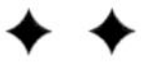

In June of 2006, I was downsized from the company I had been with for thirteen years. In my eyes and in "My Other's" (my affectionate name for my soon-to-be husband) eyes, it was a huge disappointment and relief. I started to collect unemployment. Sitting around watching TV, playing on the computer, pretty soon, my weight was inching up slowly. I could barely get in my jeans. They suffocated me to button them. I assumed I was fat and lazy. So, with the extra time, I upped my usual workout routine from 125 crunches and thirty minutes on the bike, three times a week, to 250 crunches and forty-five minutes, 4-5 days a week. The Other and I bought bikes and we made Saturday and Sunday morning ten mile rides a regular course of action on any day that Michigan weather would allow (about eight months out of the year). I helped The Other's mother with her house flipping business. I made myself move for more than ten hours a day, seven days a week. Yet that scale didn't move. It mocked me daily. The lower part of my abdomen, which had never in my life been flat, just seemed to be increasing in size especially on the sides.

My weight was met by speculation:

"You drink too much coffee 'cause you know caffeine slows down the metabolism."

"You don't drink enough water which will make you retain weight."

"You don't sleep through the night your body can't rebuild."

"Doesn't matter how many crunches you do, the fat just sits on top of the muscle."

News, TV-show doctors, internet weight-loss gurus, and friends who think they are doctors (who get their info from the internet) are plentiful. In addition, you always have interesting conversation when talking about reducing your size. This increasing lower abdomen size was easily explained (in my head) by a lifetime of not eating healthy and general laziness when it came to working out. It did not concern me in the least.

The problem with not being concerned and being downsized on top of it means no more health insurance, so I couldn't actually talk to a real doctor, unless of course you are independently wealthy. Sure there was C.O.B.R.A. I could have paid for that or my house. I chose the house. Now before you start out feeling sorry for me, I was in a decent position in my eyes. Laid off and collecting $1200 a month in unemployment, it paid most of my bills, and I had never really been sick my entire forty-three years of life. It was worth the risk in my opinion. My weight was a lifelong exercise in futility, yet there was that magic number **43**. I stopped going steadily to a doctor for my yearly doctor's visit at a critical time… pap smears, mammograms, a little blood draw. *A dangerous and possibly deadly move.* Yet, I decided: *not me.* I was invincible.

I was wrong.

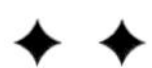

In February of 2009, three short years after my downsizing, the left gland in my neck swelled to the size of a golf ball in less than a half hour. I went to urgent care figuring it was the usual sinus infection sneaking up on me. The doctor seemed concerned that it happened so fast. He said my sinuses were inflamed and prescribed fourteen days of amoxicillin. I thought nothing of it. Sinus infections came around about once a year for me and with it, swollen glands. Nothing to be concerned over, but I point this out because nine short months later the exact same thing happened again. I went to the same urgent care and got a different doctor. He thought something was wrong and asked about any other symptoms I might be having, or things that seemed to bother me. With a doctor's ear for the price of an urgent care visit, I told him about a few things that I had been noticing. Of course, when I googled these things as they arose, all arrows pointed to menopause. So, with the self-diagnosis in my head, I thought I'd throw it out there to get a confirmation of what I thought was happening. I told this doctor about the weight gain around my stomach, my hair seemed to be thinning, insomnia, night sweats, erratic periods, and I was tired a lot. Please look at this list again. At that moment:

I was forty-six years old
Had never had children,
Had night sweats,
Insomnia,
Thinning hair,
Missed periods
And weight gain around the middle

Any woman, or man involved with a woman in her late forties or early fifties, can look at that list and say the same thing I, my friends, family, and anyone who would listen to me complain will say…

Menopause

Yep, I was positive, andalmost everyone I knew, believed it was menopause that I was going through.

When I listed these symptoms and said the word menopause to this urgent care doctor, he shook his head and said no the gland doesn't fit into the picture, and he reminded me that just a few months before, nine to be exact, I was in there for the same swollen gland, large as a golf ball, hard as a rock, and that came on in less than twenty-five minutes. Nope, he had other ideas. Epstein Barr to be exact. He prescribed amoxicillin for fourteen days telling me if the gland didn't go down he would give me a blood test to confirm his diagnosis. He also took his time and explained what Epstein Barr was. I won't go into details, but it's viral. I was shocked to learn I couldn't take a pill to get rid of it. However, the symptoms mirrored menopause, and it explained every one of them, including the gland.

Finally an answer! To my delight, and even though my symptoms screamed it, and I embraced the life style, I was *not* menopausal!

CHAPTER TWO
EXCUSES, EXCUSES

With my new found knowledge and a feeling I finally had an answer that explained all my existing symptoms, as well as the new ones, fatigue and swollen glands. I pushed through the tiredness and continued with my life. I went from sleeping six hours a night to barely getting by on nine or ten hours. I kept telling myself: *Kim you're getting older, you are no longer 25, you can't work eight hours and then come home, take care of the house, cook, and get the family ready for the next day as well as working out. This Epstein Barr is kicking your ass.* The gland went down after a few days, not completely, but good enough in my head and in the doctor's head, so he never ordered the test. I felt good and didn't want to spend the cash, so I didn't press and moved on.

I felt so happy in April of 2009 that I had finally found work, a good job, which offered insurance. Which, stupidly, I didn't take at first. I had been out of full time work for just shy of three years, and we had amassed some debt. Debt was something I wasn't used to. I had always paid my own way and didn't spend beyond my means. So being out of work for three years took its toll. I had charged to my very large credit base, taxes, groceries and gas. The Other worked fifty plus miles from home, and gas hovered at four dollars a gallon which sent what we owed up and up. I had only been making minimum payments and charging hundreds every month. I decided instead of paying the hundred and thirty dollars a month for my insurance, that I would put it toward paying down debt and pick up the insurance in about a year. I mean, so far, so good. I still had spent my life as healthy individual. I had nothing to worry about.

In May of 2009, I received devastating news. My father at age sixty-five was diagnosed with Multiple Myeloma. To put it in simple terms, bone cancer; this is a terminal cancer. I watched as the expensive treatment did a number on my parents' finances and my father's health. I thought in the mindset of: he looked and acted so much better before the chemotherapy pills were taken. It seemed as if this expensive treatment was getting the better of him. I watched a vibrant sixty-five-year-old age rapidly into a person who spent his days sleeping, laying in the recliner and his nights getting sick. We were also told treatment would be a matter of months; swallowing some forty pills in one session. What the family found out later is that you stay on the chemotherapy pills until you or your body can't take it anymore, or one of the side effects or related health issues ends your time here on earth. Never getting your life back to where it should be or ever feeling like yourself again. These are the things they do not tell you in the beginning of treatment. These were the things I wasn't listening to when I read online about the side effects and fatality rates of my dad's cancer. I breezed over article after article on what I would consider to be reputable websites: the CDC, the Cleveland Clinic, the Mayo Clinic, Karmanos, and the American Cancer Society. I was reading, but it wasn't sticking.

The severity of this vicious killer (cancer) is… and the wrath in which the 'treatment' of it takes over your life.

My dad's cancer got me thinking. He had many times told the story of his grandmother who, at about the age of sixty-five, got sick and within two years, she was dead. In the end you couldn't even touch her it was so painful. There was no way to tell but they had long suspected she had died of bone cancer. I looked at the symptoms and when they started; for most people, it was in their sixties. I read the life style reports, and symptoms, I thought I was a good candidate to watch for Multiple Myeloma in myself. In physical structure I am a lot like my dad. But I held a positive thought, if this kind of cancer is in our gene pool, what the hell sixty-five, that's not bad. Plus it was some twenty years away. I always figured me for skin cancer, some melanoma I had missed. I was constantly having skin tags and moles checked and removed. Having been a huge fan of the tanning bed in the mid 1980's, I had already had a dysplastic mole taken off of me.

Still, with all this information laid at my feet, I still wasn't concentrating on what was going on within my own body. For such an intelligent woman, I was acting like a naïve child.

In December of 2009, my long-time boyfriend asked me to marry him. Neither of us over the years had really thought much of marriage—both coming from marriages that weren't what we had hoped for. Our life had been great just the way it was, so why change it. We had been living together for ten years, and on our tenth anniversary, he proposed. I was surprised at myself and how excited and happy I was at that moment. Something that I thought we didn't want as a couple was now coming to the forefront. It was time. We were both ready and knew that we were in this together forever: it was time to make the next step.

Life moved forward quickly. Planning a wedding on a pirate ship in Las Vegas was fun, and close friends and family were also getting very excited. With that planning came the customary diet for the bride-to-be. I had gone to a friend's wedding in October. Right before that, I went to a medically supervised weight loss clinic. I had a physical and blood work done and they had me keep a diet diary for the month of October and return to the Clinic with it. They diagnosed me with a mild form of Prader Willi.

Prader Willi, the attendant told me is the feeling of always being hungry. You eat and cannot stop. People who suffer from this very rare disease usually die from complications of tremendous weight gain. When I now look up the symptoms of this disease, I know that I do not have it. The only symptom that fit is the never being satisfied with food. I don't have any of the other symptoms.

Now, I can tell you this about myself: I am always hungry. I can't remember a time of ever feeling full or satisfied with any meal. I dealt with it. I can't tell you if a blood test told them I had this illness or if it was the doctor's best guess after reading my food diary, but I had another answer to my weight gain in my lower abdomen, and as anyone who is overweight knows, all you need is an excuse for your problem. That way it is not your fault.

The doctor put me on a 'special' diet. Meant just for me, there were powders and pills, and a diet based in vegetables, fruits, and proteins with a low sodium content.

I followed that diet to the letter. And, as the first of the year and those Wedding plans rolled in, I had a support group like no other. My boss told me I was going to be a "blonde bombshell" my sisters and girlfriends constantly monitored me, and from November when I officially started that program until January my weight dropped about eighteen pounds. But my clothes still didn't fit; in particular, they did not fit around my lower abdomen. I kept thinking to myself: *this is menopause. I don't care what anyone says. This weight gain was the old-lady-bulge that I would see on other women. I just need to get more serious and try to work out more.*

I went to pick out a wedding dress, and when it came in, even though I was lighter on the scale, the dress was so tight around the middle that all of the seams had to be let out.

My Other had decided he was also going to lose a few lb's for the wedding. Not really being overweight but having put on that little stomach you start to get around forty, we thought, working out together was just the ticket.

You see, I know what everyone was thinking. You're cheating on your diet and not exercising. Yet nothing could have been farther from the truth. Let's face it, my life is not a reality show, and I am not a celebrity. I don't have four hours a day to work out. However, I do have an hour a day, and I was using it. Yet I wasn't getting any results. With him by my side, I would finally have proof that I was working out, and it wasn't working for me.

In March of 2010, the new routine was to begin. We had a bedroom in our home dedicated to my workout. It was filled with a Ski Machine, an Alpine Climber, Bike, Step, and VHS and DVD's that I had been gathering since the 1980's. I had free weights, dyna-bands, and even a heavy-bag. I was set up with music, TV, and stands to put books on to read. This was a room based on a lifetime of collecting assorted weight-loss activities. At first, The Other was a bit overwhelmed on where to start. I took the lead, excited not to have to be confined to this space by myself. I pulled out what I considered to be a fairly easy abs work-out video and a celebrity video fast forwarded to the abs section.

"This is what we'll do," I remarked confidently as I put our mats on the floor and inserted the first tape, *"We'll work on abs three nights after work for ten or fifteen minutes and we'll ride our bikes on Saturday and Sunday mornings"*

"You are still going to do more," The Other stated plainly as if he already knew the answer and was hoping the extra work outs wouldn't include him.

"Yes I'm still gonna do some stuff in the morning before work."

I started the tape and the warm up crunches began.

The Other couldn't keep up. He looked over at me pumping out crunches

"This is crazy! I can't do this! What the hell?"

He seemed genuinely bewildered.

Now, let me note here that My Other is six foot three inches tall and weighs about one-hundred and ninety-eight pounds. He plays guitar in a band in addition to a full-time job. He does the yard work and helps around this house. In other words, this is not a lazy, or in any way, out of shape man.

For the next ten minutes, he did sit-ups, not in time with the video, but he did them. I changed to the next tape, and we did ten minutes more. At the end he asked if I knew how many crunches and sit-ups I was doing.

"With both tapes 250."

He looked at me with his usual concern *"Beez (the nickname he calls me), that's not right. If you are doing these even three times a week and following your diet, your stomach should be fairly flat, not cut, but at least flat...Something's wrong"*

"Yeah." I was about to pull out one of my excuses. *"There's fat on top of those muscles."*

"You need to go to the doctors for a full physical"

"I know, but I was just checked out at that weight loss clinic. I promise I will go right after the wedding for a full physical 'cause at this job I can actually take a day or a half-day to do that and nobody will yell at me or complain."

That last statement almost cost me my life!

Growing up, I was afraid to tell my mother I was sick. I would wait and wait until I was running to the family bathroom throwing up all over with every step. Later in life, we teased my mom constantly about her being 'mean' when we were sick. She wasn't mean. She took great care of us, made us anything we wanted to eat, let us sit in my dad's recliner and watch TV all day, and usually bought us some sort of new toy to play with. I interpreted her anger in having to clean up my mess as some sort of anger directed at me as a child. It wasn't until much later in life, when I watched My Other treating his children with the exact same attitude as my own mother had. I knew for a fact that the words coming out of his mouth, weren't the same as what he was feeling. I called my mom and asked her about it. My Other being is a Virgo like my mom, and I saw in them many of the same personality traits, so I thought she could enlighten me. She was very understanding and blunt.

"I felt, and I'm sure Chris does too, that it would just be easier if WE got sick and not the kids. I couldn't fix what was wrong, and kids can't really explain things, so you don't know if they have to go to the doctor's or if it's just a little cold. It's complicated, but it is just easier to take care of yourself and never have your kids sick."

That statement made a lot of sense to me, and that evening I discussed it with Chris and he said that was exactly how he felt. I pointed out that the tone of what he was saying to his children did not reflect his caring or concern, but a strong disciplinarian. He made an effort to correct that immediately. I was happy about that and later on I ended up writing a blog about just this subject. You see, tone and intent cannot readily be interpreted by most adults and very seldom by children in such situations.

That fear that rose up in me about not wanting to make my mother 'mad at me' when I was sick filtered into my adult life. It seemed that at every job I held the fact that I went once a year to the gynecologist and twice a year to the dentist was a major problem for all of my employers. You could count the number of times on one hand that, in my twenty-three years in the field of hospitality, I called in sick, and I was given grief for it each and every time. I tried to schedule doctors/dentist visits on vacations days as to not disrupt my job, but vacation days were even met with irritability on the owner's part. The last job in hospitality I held for thirteen years, and we would get memo's constantly about when we couldn't take days off. When we did, we were made to feel guilty about it and Heaven-forbid if one of your staff did or said something in your absence because then you were in for a whole world of hurt.

My work career spanned three recessions, and I lived in constant fear of losing my job. Even though I always made my numbers, met my budgets, saved the companies money, had low employee turnover rates, it seemed there was always some overbearing, power-wielding, uncompassionate owner dangling my job like a carrot in front of me. That led to a lifetime of using urgent-care facilities and walk-in clinics instead of forming a good relationship with a doctor I liked. It was more about 'get me in the door, and get me out as quickly as possible' because there was my job I had to get back to. I had one boss back in the eighties, when I said I was going to be about two hours late for work because of a yearly check-up, he said, "no problem, take your time." I walked into work only forty-seven minutes later than usual, and he started screaming immediately about all the things that weren't done yet. Going back even further, at my first paycheck wielding job, I was fifteen years old, my parents had gone out of town, and I had gotten sick. I had a cousin who was staying with us call in sick to work for me. When I went into work three days later I was screamed at for ten minutes about 'calling in sick when my parents were out of town.' I was told "he knew" that I was out "gallivanting" with my friends... Yeah my friend the toilet... I took it, didn't say a word, and went back to my station at work when he was done yelling at me.

These types of events, like I said led to a lifetime of not forming any type of relationship with any one doctor. I thought about it many times. Wanting that 'TV show' doctor that would sit and talk to you–saying things like "I've known you a long time and..." Someone who would look out for my best interest when it came to my health. Yet, by my own admission, I never made that happen. I was outspoken when it came to so many things, yet, when it came to doctors and my own health, nothing. I knew so much medical information; reading and educating myself when family and friends became ill. I talked to my dad, who was an investigator for the Medical Examiner's office, and he gave me a world of information on the human body and its workings, and what he didn't know, he would ask the doctors. With that said, I always felt when it came to healthcare, medicines, diseases, that I was knowledgeable and up-to-date, so the lack of a primary care physician didn't bother me all that much.

Now, here was our wedding creeping up slowly, and I was not about to take any vacation days to go to the doctor now! I was working my behind off with the diet and exercise. I was also finally working full-time and managing a band part-time, there wasn't time to spend a day at a doctor's office. August was getting closer, yet my dress still wasn't fitting.

CHAPTER THREE
COWBOY UP

Things were progressing. The hotel and ceremony contracts were signed. Flights were booked for my fiancé and me as well as about 30 of our closest friends and family. This was turning into a big deal. The Other and I were overwhelmed by how happy everyone was that we were getting married. At the ten year mark, you really don't think anyone is paying attention anymore, but they were, and they were all about the fun that was to come.

Out-of-pocket, we had already spent $3500 on deposits and plane tickets, not to mention the money that my soon-to-be mother and father-in-law had given us. Our wedding present came early so we could use it to pay for part of the wedding. Plus, all of our friends had been shelling out $400 a head for plane tickets. All of this:

Nonrefundable.

✦ ✦

On June 30, 2010 my life changed.

✦ ✦

It was about 5pm. I had been home from work for a half hour. I was running the usual routine. I changed clothes, watered my flowers, and took something out for dinner. My stepson, who lives with us during the school year, had returned to his mom's house for a summer stay. Life was good. It is nice to have that carefree, no-child-in-the-house-for-a-few-weeks feeling. You don't have to worry about details like homework and milk for cereal.

I remember looking out our large front window and thinking how lucky we were. We lived in one of those post WWII bungalows, about twelve-hundred square feet if you included the attic that was turned into two bedrooms instead of the customary one. We had a very large front room window, also an unusual trait for this style of home.

I thought, *I am going to walk after dinner tonight. It is beautiful out.* Michigan gets so few perfect days, and this was one of them. Now, how could I convince The Other to do sit-ups and walk with me?

The phone rang; it was The Other. He works about fifty-five miles from our home. It's an hour plus drive in horrendous traffic. Before my downsizing I also made the same type of ride. It's trying on the temperament and the nerves. His hours had been changed from an easier ride time of 6 am and 3:30 pm to 7 am and 4:30 pm. He had to sit in the worst of it. Yet, we were both good with that. After being unemployed for three years, we were both just so thankful to be working full time and getting back on our feet.

"Hellllllooooooooooooooooo," I answered

"I'm in the car."

When you make a ride like that, they only thing that helps is distraction. Talking on the phone, listening to music; you have to or you will go nuts.

The conversation started; we've been talking like this for years, every day, for an hour while either he or I was driving from work. I grabbed a piece of paper towel and started dusting off the black ladder shelves in our living room. As the conversation progressed, I felt a little sick to my stomach. I grabbed a Diet Dr. Pepper and sat down on the couch and continued the conversation.

Soda-pop and coffee were a mainstay in my life. My blog is even subtitled under my caffeine addiction:

Kimhenderly.com

So I Age And Learn –
The Ramblings of a Caffeine Induced Mind.

Caffeine, and in particular that which comes from soda-pop, is my go-to medicine for everything. Stress, Worry, Happiness, Anger, Fatigue, and if my stomach didn't feel quite right, it is calming and soothing to me. It is also an emotional crutch at this point in my life. I can tell you on that day–June 30, 2010, my addiction to caffeine was out of control. I was consuming about two pots of coffee and at least a two liter of heavily caffeinated diet pop daily. Even my step son knew…

"Kim needs a cup of coffee" or "Where's Kim's Coke?" was a phrase heard around me all the time, and to reiterate, I was now sleeping 9-10 hours a day. Caffeine was my lifeline to get done all I needed to accomplish in an average day.

I sat down on the couch that sunny, Michigan, early evening, talking about our days and sipping my drink. I moved to put my feet up on the couch and lean against its padded arm. I looked and my shoes were on, and I thought to myself, if The Other were home he'd be yelling at me.

"Ok, I just got off the expressway. Be there soon. Love you!"

"London Broil for dinner! Love you too!"

I clicked the end button on the phone, set the phone down on the coffee table, and went to swing my feet down to the floor to get up off the couch. A pain shot through my left lower abdomen, almost at the pelvic region.

"DAMMIT!" I shouted. *"What the hell is that?!"* I thought. I couldn't move my feet to the floor it was so painful. I tried to lift the top of my body with my arms by pushing off the couch. Still the same pain. I was paralyzed into that feet-up position.

I was completely confused. Did I pull a muscle? Get a cramp? Have to go to the bathroom? No matter which way I moved, I had severe pain in the same spot. I looked up at the screen door. It was locked. Even when The Other came home, he wouldn't be able to get in the house to help me without wrecking the door. I was screwed. I sat there for five minutes watching the wind blow threw the silver maple tree across the street and breathed deeply, hoping beyond hope that this was some fluke, and it would pass. Distraction, I needed to think of something else. I turned on the television and flipped through the channels. Five more minutes passed, and I went to move my legs again, the pain was worse, and now it was starting to hurt even just sitting there. I shut off the TV and took a last deep breath.

"Ok Kim, you can do this. It's only going to hurt for a minute, and then you will be up."

With everything I had, I swung my legs to the floor and pushed myself upward using the coffee table. I got up, and the pain was so bad my knees buckled, and I fell to the floor wedged between the coffee table and the couch.

"Awe hell no!" I pushed the coffee table away, and I crawled to the front door on all fours to unlock it and then back to the couch and waited for The Other's arrival.

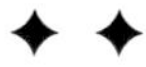

He came in the front door and smiled. *"Hi Beez!"*

I started to feel better because I knew he was close. I made my best sad face. *"My side hurts."*

"Do you need to poop?" If nothing, he's blunt.

"I don't think so."

"Do you need to go to the doctors?" He asked with the irritation rising in his voice (there was that childhood fear creeping in, telling someone I was sick and their irritation with me). I remembered my mom's words and tried to analyze my words before I blurted them—for some reason I knew this time was different and I couldn't cover up an illness and go on with life as usual.

I knew that my statement of "my side hurts" was not the normal or planned evening he was used to. I would need to tell him an exactly what was wrong and how I was going to handle it, and if I needed his help, I would have to be specific about what that need was. There was one problem, I didn't know, and had no experience in my life to draw from to answer the questions he was going to have.

My eyes started to tear up. I was not a big crier at that point in my life, but I was scared.

"I don't know?...No"

"Well which is it?" He says neatly putting away his lunch box and its contents.

"Come here."

He came and sat on the couch next to me.

"I'm scared. This really hurts. I couldn't even get off the couch."

"Once again," He said firmly, *"Do you need to go to the doctor's?"*

"Yes, but I can't take time off work. We just lost an employee and besides I can't go to urgent care. Where am I going to go? I don't have a regular doctor." I was rambling out of fear.

"Let's call my mom."

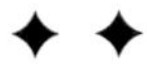

Enter my soon to be mother-in-law, Sue. She was forced into early retirement and had what neither of us had: time.

I called and explained what was wrong, how I didn't want to miss work, and couldn't call around at work to find a doctor. She said she would take care of it. The good thing was it was Wednesday, and I was off on Friday for the Fourth of July holiday. I was hoping for a Friday appointment, so I wouldn't miss any work. Over the years I had done something very stupid. I put my jobs in front of everything important in my life. I was leaning in that same stupid direction again. However, turning it over to someone that I trusted, and I knew had recent experience in finding good doctors for friends made me feel better. Like a burden of fear had been lifted from me.

I spent that evening hunched over my computer looking up symptoms. Everything was coming up Kidney Stones. The good thing about the internet is you can find out anything. The bad thing about the internet is there is no filter, no 'for sure', it is a hodge-podge, even on reputable sites of information, that at best, only partially relate to you. I read for the next three hours. Then I lay in bed on my side, propping what had now become my enormous stomach up with pillows. It was like the sheer weight of my stomach was causing the pain. *You stupid fat ass!* I thought to myself, *you brought this on yourself with all this weight gain!*

I stared at the TV by the reflection in the picture hanging on the wall and started to think. I used to sleep on my back. Always, when did that stop? A year ago? Two? The weight from my stomach had made it impossible for me to lie on my back; I've taught myself how to sleep on my side. I felt around my stomach. This must weigh thirty pounds. This is why I have to pee every ten minutes, all this pressure on my bladder, forget what the doctors said... several years ago, when I was thirty-five at an annual gynecologist visit, I had made mention of my frequent urination. Pills were just becoming available to help with these types of problems. I thought I might have needed some pills to help with the frequent urination problems. He said it was far more likely I had a 'pinched bladder' that I was too young for frequent urination problems. With that thought in my head... was it TEN YEARS ago when it started? Here is one of those problems, because I didn't see the same doctor every year, or even go into the same doctor's office, there was no record of any question or concern I raised, no follow up on anything. In fact, I never brought up the frequent urination again. I blamed it on the 'pinched bladder.' "SBS," I used to joke with my friends, "small bladder syndrome," –my girlfriend coined that phrase saying she thought her husband had the same thing. We were both always peeing!

It was too much to think about, and now I was lying in bed over analyzing every single detail that had gone on with me physically for the past decade, yet I seemed to have an excuse for everything that went wrong over the years. All the excuses and statements lead to the same thing... I was overweight. Now, as I lay there trying to get comfortable, I thought about someone I knew who had passed several kidney stones and the narcotics they had given him for pain. I didn't want to go through that, yet I had such a feeling of doom I just *knew* that was coming.

Little did I know that I completely missed the mark.

CHAPTER FOUR

KIDNEY STONES, THE LESSER OF TWO EVILS

The Other's mom had gotten me an appointment the next day. It was Thursday July 1, 2010; the appointment was at 2:15. I thought to myself… well I can work most of the day. I had been leaving work at 3:30pm daily by not taking a lunch hour so I could be home for my stepson, a habit I had picked up watching another girl in the office do the same thing. My boss didn't seem too upset at all by the fact that I was taking off almost an hour early to see a doctor about a pain in my side. They were pushing me out the door to be on time. This was a novelty for me. In my former profession, I would have been met with great resistance to taking off even five minutes early. It just wasn't done: there were no holidays off, or paid sick days. You worked sick or not. So to hear someone say out loud *"shouldn't you be on your way to the doctors"* was not only amazing to me, but it took a major stress off me. I thought that perhaps being sick with a kidney stone wouldn't be the total loss of my job. A job that I had fallen in love with, because it was so different from anything that I had ever done.

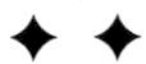

Sue picked me up at my house fifteen minutes before the appointment, as she drove she asked me: *"What do you think you have?"*

"I was reading a lot on the computer last night. Gosh, I hope it's not kidney stones" (Now who would have thought that kidney stones would have been the lesser of two evils!)

She replied, *"Well whatever it is, I want you to go in there and act really sick. You get farther with these people when you pretend like you are in a lot of pain."*

The pain… you remember… the pain that wouldn't allow me to get off the couch less than twenty-four hours ago… it was there, and here was another general problem with me… working through the pain. In my world, I call that 'cowboying up'–*"work through that pain, don't be a baby, suck it up, go to work, take care of your business, only whiners and complainers lay around in pain."* Hence the reason I was now being driven to a doctor's appointment that I didn't make. My Other knew me well enough to know that I wouldn't have made the appointment or gone to the doctors on my own. I would have sucked it up. After all, I had managed to get up off that couch eventually, make dinner, do a little internet doctoring, watch TV, get up in the morning make lunches and go to work. All with a paralyzing pain, that *I was now starting to adapt to.*

When we reached the medical building for one of the major hospital centers in the area, my mother-in-law dropped me at the door and as I exited her car she told me, *"Look sick and go sit on that bench."* I did. When she walked up, she stood in front of the automatic doors waited for them to open and then loudly said, *"Do you need a wheel chair?"* The statement was for the benefit of anyone within ear shot. *"No I'm ok."* We walked in and I followed her to the elevator. Sue kept asking as we passed medical personnel, *"Do you need a wheelchair?"* The statement would make people turn and look at me. I was walking slowly with almost a limp type step and holding my side, I hadn't realized that I had probably been doing that all day.

When we got to the correct suite, I looked at the name on the door. Damn, I had seen this doctor in 2002 after moving from the northern suburbs to the downriver area, he was an ass. I only went to him once, and he seemed very concerned with promoting his own agenda and the products he liked as opposed to doing what I wanted. At the time, I was looking for a new doctor, so I wouldn't have to drive over an hour to see the gynecologists (yes plural) on the other side of town. It was one of those moments that I mentioned, that I felt maybe I should have a 'regular doctor,' someone I could go to all the time. He was down the street from my home and I realized walking in that this was his second office. He was affiliated with a well-known hospital in

2002, and judging by the sign outside by the street, he had maintained that relationship. When I saw him the first time in '02, I asked for a refill on my birth-control pills. He wanted me to have surgery to input a new little experimental device that had been out since 2000 (now known as Mirena). It sounded like an IUD, and I wasn't interested. He spent twenty minutes trying to convince me otherwise. He never even finished the exam on me, just left in a huff and had the nurse bring in the Rx for my pills. Well, I concluded, that was seven years ago, maybe he's changed. I mentioned to my mother-in-law that, *"I thought I recognized the name."* She quickly said, *"Oh you're seeing the nurse practitioner. I couldn't get you in with the doctor."* I was relieved.

I was called in not long after my check-in and paperwork were completed. The nurse herself walked me back, gave the usual instructions on disrobing and said she would be back. When she re-entered the room she sat down and asked, *"Why are you here today?"* No doctor had ever asked me that question before. Usually they looked at the quick notes an aide wrote down, did an exam, diagnosed, and I was on my way. I liked it like that. Quick. In and Out. Done.

I said to the nurse *"I had a pain in my side."*

"Can you elaborate on that?"

I paused and in a second I had sized up this woman. An over achiever who wanted to be a doctor without putting in the time. The only other time I had seen a nurse practitioner, she would only write me a Rx for birth-control for six months so I had to come back and pay for a second exam that year. I wasn't impressed.

I relayed exactly what had happened to this woman, adding the fact that I am a very active person. I have to say things like this. It is my own personal validation for those who don't know me. I am not some oversized woman who sits on her ass watching TV and complaining; I have a very full, very active lifestyle. Do I run five miles a day? Nope, but on a good day, I can physically out-work the most fit person fifteen years younger than me. She looked at me with doubt in her ever judging eyes.

"OK Kim, I need you to lie back on the exam table."

"Yeah, I can't lie on my back it hurts." I figured I would play it up a little like Sue had told me to.

The nurse practitioner grabbed my hand and helped me lie back. She did a very thorough digital exam and then removed her gloves extended her hand and arm for me to grab and pulled me into an upright position.

"Um." There were those judging eyes again. "You know what," she paused, *"Get dressed and we'll talk."* The sarcastic tone in her voice made me immediately wonder, *what the hell is going on? Just flippin' tell me!*

"Ok, it won't take me long." My way of letting this woman know not to leave me sitting here forever. As the door closed softly behind her, I couldn't help but think that this must be something really stupid judging by her look and tone. Like some menopausal period cramps, but that feeling didn't last long.

I hadn't realized with everything on my mind and the day of work how bad the pain was actually becoming. I had a hard time redressing myself. The easy task of slipping into a pair of dress pants required me to sit on a chair, instead of the usual stand and lift a leg into the pants. I felt like a little kid who knows the physicality of dressing but is slow and awkward carrying out the task.

The nurse opened the door as I slipped on my second patent leather pump. She looked down at my shoes and commented on how 'nice' they were. She was trying to be a different person with me. Softer, quieter, less irritated and judgmental.

"Kim, do you have insurance?" she said in her nicest voice

I was pissed, and I snapped back, *"What the hell difference does that make?! Is there a problem?! Is this all in my head?! Am I just too fat and having pains because of it?!"*

"Kim, what do you think is wrong?"

Really? This is what we are doing? Playing twenty questions?

"If I knew I wouldn't be here, but if you are asking my opinion I thought I might have a kidney stone or maybe a gallbladder issue, do I win?" I tried not to sound too mean, but I couldn't help the sarcasm and irritability that was coming out.

"You're not a regular patient here so I don't have a full medical back ground on you..." Her voice trailed off.

"Ask me anything you need to know, I've got nothing to hide!" I

spewed out sharply

"Do you have children?"

"I have two step-children. One lives with us full time; one does not. Why?"

"So you couldn't have children?"

"NOOOOO, I was selfish when I was younger, and I much preferred expensive purses, shoes and travel." I said as I extended out the shoe she had commented on, hoping that she would know that they cost well over $100.

"So I noticed that in your paperwork that you filled out today you wrote down that you were menopausal: Who told you that?"

"A doctor! Get to the point, do you know what's causing the pain or not?!"

"Kim," she got a very large smile *"You are about 22 weeks pregnant!"*

"NO I'M NOT!" I said loudly and defiantly.

"Yep, I felt a baby, and by the size, I would say you are pretty far along. As for the pain I think the baby is putting pressure on..."

I cut her off mid-sentence, *"Hey, listen to me. I am 47 years old. I know how to use birth-control; I am not pregnant."* I know I must have looked appalled by the thought of being pregnant, but it wasn't that I didn't want to be pregnant. If I was ever going to have a child, it would have been with My Other. I knew that we practiced safe sex and we had no malfunctions in the last few months.

The nurse practitioner leaned back in her chair to reach into a drawer. She pulled out a stick wrapped in the commercial plastic. I had seen these before, I had used one a year ago when I missed my first period, and hence had convinced myself that I was menopausal.

She handed it to me *"The restroom is right across the hall, leave it sitting on the sink; don't put it in the door like the instructions on the wall say."*

"Ok." I grabbed the stick and went across the hall to pee on the stick. I set the pregnancy test on the wrapper and set it down on the sink. As I exited the rest room, the nurse came out of the exam room.

"Were you able to urinate enough?"

I quipped, *"I can pee anywhere at any time."*

She grabbed the stick with a gloved hand and sat back down in the exam room with me.

"This will only take a few seconds" she paused *"huh??"* a quizzical sound came from her.

"What does it say?"

"Well…" There was another dramatic long pause…*"You're not pregnant,"* she said flatly.

"No shit, now what?"

"Well I felt something. I am going to send you for a trans-vaginal ultrasound."

Another test, *another* day off work, I was irritated *"Where do I have to go for that?"*

"We can do it right here. Right now."

Jumping at the chance to handle this, I remarked *"Let's do this."*

"I also want to get some blood from you."

"Sure, can I do that here?"

"Yes."

Now the reality set in. She had felt something, so I had to inquire, *"What do you think you felt?"*

"Let's wait for the ultrasound."

"Best guess?" I pushed.

"Some type of tumor, but let's look at the ultrasound results first."

I was led around a corner and four doors down.

"Undress from the waist down and have a seat." And with that, the door closed.

Great undress again! I was pissed. As I sat on the table with my paper blanket, the door opened and a twenty-something pretty girl entered the room. She introduced herself and asked if I had ever had a trans-vaginal ultrasound? I replied no, and she showed me the wand she would be inserting in me to take a look around. I had to ask why they couldn't do it from the outside like they do for babies. She explained how this would give them a much better look at all the female pieces.

As she inserted the wand, which looked like an extra-large white vibrator with a big round ball on the end; the tech hit a button on the computer screen, and I heard her gasp.

"What do you see?" I turned my head and looked at the screen. It

was black except for some small words around the edges.

"Umm... I'll let you talk to the nurse. Hold still. Just a few more pictures."

"Seriously, what did you see?"

She removed the wand and gave me instructions on getting dressed and returning to the exam room, never giving me a chance to ask again what she saw. She quickly left the room and shut the door.

I dressed myself in the sitting position and found my way back to the exam room I had been in. The nurse practitioner appeared almost immediately. She sat across from me and started talking.

"You have a large mass. I don't know what it is but it's at least 22cm. It covers so much area that we can't tell where it's coming from. The ovaries? The uterus? I want to have the doctor look at it. He will be here in about an hour. You can go have blood drawn, and I want to do a CA125 with that blood work, then if you want you can come back to the waiting room, and I will talk to the doctor when he gets here and maybe we will have more answers." She talked so fast. Gone was the judgment, the happiness, the professional bedside manor had kicked in. Just the facts, don't give anything away.

"Ok, where do I go to do the blood and what is a CA125?"

"Downstairs in the lab"

"... and the CA125?"

"You've never had one?"

"Nope."

"Wait, didn't you put that your grandmother and aunt had cancer?" She inquired as she reached for my file and started flipping pages.

"Yes, my grandmother had ovarian at age 83, and her sister had breast cancer."

"And nobody has ever ordered a CA125 or a trans-vag?"

"Nope"

"Have you told your doctors this information?"

"Yep, every one of them," and of course by that I meant the dozens of doctors I had seen over the years. Every time you go to a new office they make you fill out those forms, and every time I wrote down my grandmother and her sister both had cancer. Some doctors even mentioned it to me to confirm the cancer, what type, and that it was on my dad's side of the family.

"Oh for…." Her voice trailed off. *"A CA125 measures levels of cancer antigens. It is not a perfect test, but it is the only thing we've got. Higher numbers combined with other information could give you an early warning for certain cancers. Of course we get a lot of false positives on this test. A cold could make the numbers high, but I think you should have it done."*

"Okay, I agree."

She walked me to the waiting room and explained how to get to the lab.

I talked to Sue on the way down and told her every detail. The good thing about me is that I can recall conversations and events in great detail, a trait I've had since childhood. A memory like a vault, details retained for years and years. Chris's mom got upset, having just lost a friend to a cancer that had gone undiagnosed until she was at death's door.

The blood work was uneventful as was the wait for the doctor to come in. I called My Other, who was working and told the detailed story again to him. The nurse called for me to come back, and we returned to the same exam room.

"The doctor doesn't know what this is. He recommends you find a general surgeon and have this mass removed A.S.A.P."

"Wait …. What? That's it? You got a name, a place to call? What kind of surgery?"

"I don't really have any answers except for what I've told you, you can see the girls at the desk on the way out. Good luck" and with that she left the room.

Surgery? Mass? Go somewhere else? What the hell was going on?

I walked mindlessly to the girls at the desk. Better pay that co-pay! The check-out was over $300. It was late in the day, late in the week on a holiday that was fast approaching. I was too stunned and too much of an idiot to argue. I handed over my credit card.

CHAPTER FIVE

THE FIRST INKLINGS THAT I WAS IN OVER MY HEAD

I was off the next day for the holiday weekend, and I woke up and started calling 'general surgeons.' Nobody would see me. Not one. I was at a loss. I started to inquire among my nurse friends. One name came up over and over. This was the guy I wanted to go after.

My mother-in-law went to his office personally and got me an appointment on Tuesday July 5th after work. I was feeling better until a call came in that day after lunch. It was the nurse practitioner from the Doctor's office, she had the lab results.

"Your CA125 is 1442."

"What does that mean?"

"It is supposed to be under 35."

"AGAIN WHAT DOES THAT MEAN?" I screamed into the phone, tired of not getting a direct answer.

"Well with the mass it could be cancer. That number is really high."

"And the false positives?" I asked hoping.

"Probably not, but good news, I found a place for you to call – the Wayne County Women's Clinic."

"Do they do surgery?" I asked.

"No."

"Then what good does that do me?" I asked irritated.

"Well maybe they can guide you."

"To what?"

"Find someone."

"Isn't that what you were supposed to do?" I hung up on her.

It was Friday July 2, 2010, and this is what I knew:

I had a mass of over 22cm (that is about 9 inches). Get a piece

> of paper and hold the short side up to your stomach. Now I knew why I couldn't lose any weight in my lower abdomen! That is quite large.
>
> I also knew that my markers for possible cancer were 1442 and were supposed to be under 35.
>
> I also knew I had to sit with that information for the next four days.... Actually it was one-hundred and two hours. I knew that wouldn't work for me so I started researching....

I called the 800 number for the American Cancer Society, and told the volunteer who answered the phone my tale as she listened patiently. She spoke slowly, softly, and confidently after I had told her everything:

"Ok, don't panic. What I am going to do for you because I think you have very specific medical questions you need answered is I am going to have one of our oncology nurses call you back, is that ok?"

"Yes."

"Can I get a number you can be reached at within the next hour?" She politely asked.

"Sure." As I gave her my number I couldn't help but think, *why isn't anyone answering my specific questions?*

I hung up the phone and less than five minutes later a nurse called back. She took the time to explain a trans-vaginal ultrasound and what it shows, and what the doctors look for. Then she explained CA125s what causes false positives and what does not. She said she couldn't tell me what kind of cancer I had, only a doctor trained in that field could and then she advised me to go to the doctor's office I had been to and get all the records they had to take on my first visit to my next doctor. I thanked her and hung up the phone. She was fairly certain, but couldn't confirm that I had some sort of gynecological cancer. So I picked up the phone and did what most people do from this area. I called one of the most well know cancer hospital in the area at their 800 number.

The girl who answered the phone asked,

"Do you have a diagnosis?"

"No."

I recounted my story of what happened. She said I needed a diagnosis to get one and call back. I asked another question and she quipped, *"We are not a question and answer line"* My future mother-in-law called back and tried a different approach saying she had reports and ultrasounds and managed to get an appointment for July 14th at 10am. As she hung up the phone she said, *"We'll use that as a back-up if the doctor on the 6th doesn't work out."*

I was angry. This was the biggest and best cancer center in the area!! Sue had managed to get me an appointment by lying and saying we had 'results' when really we didn't.

I would come to learn in the coming months many, many things. The biggest being that even though I was a well-read individual and considered myself to be fairly intelligent... and even though I knew many people who had cancer, including my own father, and other assorted family members... and even though I had read books, watched movies about chemotherapy and its side-effects...

I knew nothing about cancer, <u>its treatment</u>, life expectancy or any other part of the disease.

If you would have asked me before July 2, 2010 if I knew about cancer, it's treatments and life expectancy I would have told you, *"Sure, you'd have to be living under a rock to not know."* Well on that day I personally crawled out from under that same rock, put on a pair of glasses to block the sun and dusted myself off.

All so that cancer could slap me hard back down to the ground.

CHAPTER SIX
THE LONGEST WEEKEND

That Fourth of July weekend in 2010 was the longest and the shortest in my entire life. I fretted and worried. I talked and discussed. I researched and read. My Other, being very worried had tried to keep the weekend 'normal.' We attended an annual Fourth of July party at my BFFs home. It helped that there were additional nurses at the party. I got their opinions and everyone tried being as positive as they could. The worry and the stress that goes with a tiny bit of knowledge but no answers never went away. In my case, all I wanted to do was talk about it and tell people about what happened at the doctor's office. I know Chris got sick of hearing the story of the pregnancy diagnosis and the rude treatment from all the places I called, but I didn't care. It kept it fresh in my mind and the more I talked about it, the more it became a story and the less it was about me suffering with this tumor.

I wore a very flowing shirt as I had been for months to hide my lower abdomen. Trying to be me; I really needed someone to jump in a conversation at some point and say, *"oh hey, I know someone, and it was no big deal this, and this takes place,"* but that never happened. No matter how many people I told the story to, nobody even spoke up about whether or not they had or knew anyone who had cancer. Everyone just listened, all weekend long. To my story.

Chris kept reassuring me that everything was going to be ok. We would go to the doctors on Tuesday; they would tell us what's wrong, and then it would be taken care of and be fine. Yet, I had my doubts.

My closest friend Charlotte, a year earlier, had a medical issue. I got a call early on a Saturday morning from her then fiancé saying she had been checked into the hospital the night before. I high-tailed it with The Other in tow to see her. She explained the double pulmonary embolism and what had happened the night before that lead to her admittance to the hospital. Had she not been a nurse, I would be writing a very different paragraph about her right now. I bring it up because after she explained all the medical jargon, I looked at her and said:

"So what do they do for this surgery? Just cut them right out since they caught them? Or meds to shrink them?"

"They can't do anything."

"What?" I was floored. *"What do you mean they can't do anything? This is America! We have the greatest healthcare system in the world! You don't have some rare disease. You have an embolism, THAT YOU CAUGHT IN TIME! Most people drop dead from these things! What do you mean there is no treatment!"*

The conversation went on from there with me, Chris, Charlotte and Sean discussing American healthcare and the country's interpretation of 'we can do anything'.

We can't.

It was an eye-opener and I had carried that thought through the weekend, that doctors can't fix everything, yet the years of my beliefs that in America we fix all illnesses with the right doctor, hospital, and most of all money, started to take over. I pushed my initial response of 'oh no poor me' right out of my head, and by the time I went to work on Tuesday, I was back to: *'In America we fix all!'*

I worked the entire day at my job letting the owner of my company know what had happened at the doctor's and letting her know about my 6 pm appointment. I played it off like it was no big deal.

I had fully adapted to the pain in my side for work. It bothered me more when I had nothing else to focus on. I was busy at work so it was tolerable.

I headed out the door on my way home for Sue to pick me up to go to this new doctor's office. Late office hours, I like that. With My Other heading home from work also, we were in touch and I was hoping that he wouldn't hit any major traffic malfunctions on the way. Thankfully we all pulled into the parking garage of the hospital within minutes of each other. Once again, Sue started with the *"do you need a wheelchair"* and *"act really sick."* I was good until we walked off the elevator into the hospital and I saw in four foot letters across the bricks: CANCER CENTER. The absolute reality of it all hit me when I saw that sign.

Cancer.

I knew it could be, yet I had talked myself out of it over the weekend. Quite frankly, had it not been for My Other and his mom physically making me go to these appointments, I wouldn't be writing this right now. I would have avoided and worked through the pain; I would have lived and worked until I keeled over.

The doctor's office was directly across from the large letters on the wall. As Chris held the door open, I walked through the entrance, and I noticed how incredibly small the waiting room was compared to most doctors' offices I had been in. There were only a dozen or so chairs in the triangular waiting room with only four chairs on one of the walls next to a cart with graham crackers, water, juice, and coffee. I walked up the woman at the reception desk.

"Hi, I'm Kim, I have an appointment." I said with hesitation. I was horrible at remembering names.

"Hi Kim," she smiled and handed me the obligatory clipboard. *"Fill this out and bring it back up with your ID and insurance info."*

When I sat down with Chris and his mom, it left no chairs open. It was 5:30 pm. We were exactly the half an hour early that they had requested to fill out forms. I filled out everything and watched as people were called back. I noticed as most of them went back with another person: husband, daughter, mother. I handed in my forms and read the information about the doctor that was available around the office. I also at that point was learning what 'gynecological oncologist' meant. The doctor I was about to see fell into that category. According to one of the ladies at work, and many nurses that I knew, if you needed a gynecological surgery this was the guy to see. There was a framed news article from an in-hospital periodical with his picture and a brief biography. He was a handsome man, and he looked like a TV-show doctor. I smiled when I thought about that, I had always wanted a TV-show doc; let's see if he lives up to the high standard that television brings. A nearly impossible task, almost like woman trying to live up to the pearls and high heel housecleaning and cooking June Cleaver.

I watched the clock tick away 6, 6:15, 6:25.... People kept arriving and people kept getting called back however, they exited at a very slow pace. I was getting impatient. I pointed out the time to Chris who whispered back:

"They fit you in. Relax."

I thought to myself, *if they don't call me by 6:30, I'm leaving,* as soon as the thought hit my head, the door opened, and a middle-aged woman called my name out. Chris and I followed her through the door.

She weighed me, took my blood pressure and put me in a room. As Chris sat in the chair and I sat on the table, we talked once again about what I could have. He tried to reassure me that we would have answers in moments from now. A woman entered the room and introduced herself as the doctor's fourth year resident; she was also a doctor. Because I knew so many people in the medical field, I knew she was probably only months away from actually being on her own. She read everything I wrote on the forms and told me to tell her why I was here. I recanted the story; she had The Other step out, so she could do an exam. When Chris came back in, she said the doctor would be in in a few moments to go over details, but basically they would go in, take out the mass and do exploratory work in the entire abdomen to see where this is coming from.

"Is this cancer?" I asked flatly. *"A friend who is a radiologist thought it might be a fibroid because it is so large."*

She nodded her head silently in the yes fashion, *"Your CA125 is very high. We won't know for sure 'til the doctor opens you up but more than likely. Do you have children?"*

There was that stupid question again, *"I have two step children."*

"Were you planning on having any children?"

Yes at close to age 50 I was going to start a family! What was wrong with these medical people? I held my sarcastic tone and answered her:

"No, why?"

"Because we will probably have to take the uterus, we could leave the ovaries so you don't go into menopause..."

"Oh hell no! If you are gonna open me up, take it all. I'm not going to

be sitting back here in two years with someone saying 'now we have to go back in and take the ovaries,' that's just stupid."

"Ok, that will send you into menopause."

"I've been having menopausal symptoms for a while; I can handle it."

I noticed Chris moving next to me. He was positioning himself on the floor I knew the routine–he thought he was going to pass out. Damn-it. I was irritated. The resident focused her attention on Chris.

"Are you ok?" She asked with concern.

"He's going to pass out." I said as The Other said, *"I'll be fine in a minute."*

"Can I get you some juice or some crackers?"

"That would be great," I answered on his behalf.

The resident left the room, finally I had someone talking to me in an intelligent fashion, and she was gone. I was beyond angry.

"This is why I don't come to the doctor."

"I'll be fine in a minute."

"Did you eat before you came?" Chris had a habit of going long periods of time if I didn't stay on him, of not eating. Which in the best of circumstances will cause him to have headaches and get light-headed; add stress, bad news or things not going his way, and passing out was almost certain. My guess was he ate somewhere around 11 am, and now it was going on 7 pm.

"It's just that you talk so graphically about all this medical stuff." He said trying to take deep breaths.

The door opened and the aide walked in with juice and graham crackers and handed them to Chris who was now back in the chair. He drank the juice and ate the crackers.

"Do you need to wait in the lobby with your mom or step out and get some air? I need to be able to talk details with the doctor."

He agreed and went to the waiting room. As I was told later, he sat down and told his mom it was cancer.

A few minutes later the resident walked in with my soon-to-be-new doctor. He was tall and thin with a beautiful smile. He walked in confidently and shook my hand with both of his and said,

"It is a privilege and an honor to meet you Kimberly."

"Kim."

"Ok, Kim, so you've met with my resident, and she told you all the facts. Large mass and you've probably got cancer. Well, I don't think you do. Lay back on the table for me." He felt around the outside of my abdomen and commented. "See how this moves and is solid?"

"Yeah."

"I think it's an out of control fibroid."

A huge sense of relief filled me up, as the doctor went on to say:

"Fibroids grow rapidly and out of control and can get very large in a very short period of time."

"What about the CA125? It's so high."

"Not really, they can get into the tens of thousands but the number is high and a fibroid can cause that. I looked at what your history is. I just don't see it. Now I've been wrong before. Nobody's perfect. Ask these women around the office. They tell me every day every little thing I do wrong."

And there it was…My TV-show doctor repertoire that I always wanted! I was so happy to have this guy as my doctor, but my train of thought was interrupted:

"Now we do have to open you up this is major surgery. I can't get to it any other way. So, do you have kids?"

"No, I already told the resident. Take it all."

"So we're taking ALL the goodies?" he said with all seriousness, and I knew on his part this is the stuff he is required to do and say by hospital regulation.

"Yes."

"Do you want to leave the ovaries so you don't go into menopause? You probably have another seven years before you should start menopause."

"No, I'm not doing this twice. Take it all." And then it was my turn to get serious, *"Listen Doc, I don't want to do this twice, and I mean that. So I know you know what cancer looks like, you know what it smells like, so if you get in there and you see anything, you take it and whatever it is attached to. You don't need to wake me up and get my permission to go back in. Do it while I'm on the table. Anything. Anywhere. OK?"*

Charlotte had told me that they know when they open you up; cancer is black and it smells. With that knowledge at my disposal, I needed to make sure this guy knew that I knew what the surgery was all about, and I wasn't going through this multiple times. The doc spoke up:

"I got it, and while I am there, I will check around everywhere. We will do the exploratory and make sure you are clean, but I'm telling you, I really think you are." He took my hand. *"Now I know you have people waiting for you out there. Let's bring them in. I want to make sure I answer everyone's questions. You got me for as long as you need me."* He really was unbelievable, and I was no longer upset about the long wait. He fit me in and he is taking his time. Wow, just like on TV. I was captivated.

As he was saying that, the resident stuck her head out the door and by the time he finished up his sentence Chris and his mom were walking through the door. My new doctor introduced himself and shook both their hands. Chris's mom was already crying, the doctor said:

"You ok?"

She nodded yes.

He repeated what he thought I had and what he was going to do and then asked for questions.

"How soon can we do this?" I asked.

"I'm in the office on Tuesdays, and I do surgery on Wednesdays here. Unless you live out by Pontiac, I can do it out there on a different day. But the girls they handle all that. I'm not allowed 'cause I mess things up. They will tell you all the dates."

"When can I go back to work?"

"You are going to be in the hospital after the surgery for 4-7 days. We like to get you out fast because we don't want you to catch anything, but you are going to be off work for 4-8 weeks." ...And then I heard it for the first time, ***"Everybody's different."***

I bought into that line, and went with *everyone's different*. I knew that when it came to illness that I rebounded faster than anyone I knew. Pain didn't bother me. After all I had a wisdom tooth removed, ended up with dry socket, and sucked it up and never took any additional pain killers. I worked through the pain. Piece of cake...I already had it figured out in those split seconds, three days in the hospital, four weeks on the couch and I'd be back to work. I would use up my vacation time, take a few unpaid weeks and be back to it.

I continued my questions, *"Can I work from home?"*

"What do you do?"

"I work on a computer."

"Sitting all day?"

"Yep."

"Sure you can work from home as soon as you want."

Sue piped in and was now in full blown tears *"So it's not cancer?"*

Great! We were back on that?

"I don't believe so." The doctor patiently turned to talk to Sue.

"We'll go in and take out everything by Kim's request, so she doesn't have to worry about this again."

I butted in, *"I told them to look around if they find anything to take it and all it touches. They don't have to wake me up to ask permission. Take it all ovaries, uterus, etc."*

Sue looked at the doctor. *"What's the difference if you leave like the uterus?"*

Knowing I understood and she was having a hard time he looked at me and smiled and winked then looked at Sue. *"About $500."* He and I laughed while Sue continued to cry.

This was also starting to irritate me. This visit was supposed to be all about me. I had a great doctor and a fabulous resident, and this crying was starting to pull focus again.

"So what can I expect after the surgery?" I interrupted again. The answer I got was probably the biggest understatement that had ever been uttered to me. That along with the fact that I personally am an idiot and think everything medical is *no big deal* would soon create the perfect storm.

"Well you're going to be sore for a while but it will pass. We will get you some pills. You will come see me a few weeks later. If you need anything you call the office. So do you want to do this WITH ME?" Wow, he was asking my opinion. I realized he was letting me know I could get a second opinion, and he wouldn't be offended.

"YES!" I had made up my mind while sitting there that I wasn't going to wait for another doctor to hear a similar diagnosis, if I could even get one to see me in a timely fashion. This guy's office had fit me in following a holiday weekend, and it was obvious, that the office was busy!

He walked over to me and took my hands in his again, "*The girls will set up your appointments. If you don't have any more questions... Kimberly it has been an honor and a privilege. Don't worry I will take care of you!*" He turned and asked if there was anything at all that anybody wanted to talk about, and I said no even though he was looking at Chris and his mom. He patted Sue on the shoulder and said it is going to be fine and with that he left the room. Another woman came in with a calendar with dates and times. The surgery would take place in eight days. They thought about getting me in the next day but by the time we got done with the doctor it was almost 7:30 and there was no way to set it up.

Trying to fit in a major surgery the very next day should have sent up all kinds of warning flags with me. However, it didn't. I, in my totally planned existence, now had a full week to make arrangements and take care of every detail.

The woman I had spoken to at the front desk gave instructions on where to go to give blood, where to call for instructions for the surgery along with the days and times to do that. She let me know that someone would call me the day before the surgery with further instructions. I liked this. In fact, it was telling me that this was my dream doctor's office. I didn't have to make any appointments or call anyone–two things I was terrible at–they did everything right there for me and gave me a list. Perfect. This was going to be so easy!

What an incredibly stupid thing to think!

With the relief of what the doctor said, I felt great. The pain was only noticeable when I slept or thought about it. I worked it out with my job for vacation days and unpaid time off, and they didn't yell, complain or make me feel guilty like all my past places employment. Actually they were very supportive and helpful. When I said I was going to work the day before the surgery, the owner insisted I take the day off to center myself. Alright, I didn't feel I needed to, but I took it to be alone with my thoughts, and to prepare the house and myself for post-surgery. The Other put in for a week and a half of vacation time. Figuring surgery on the following Wednesday and the remainder of that week, followed by the whole next week, by then I would be home and settled. If I needed help after those eleven days, my mom and dad or his mom could come by and help. We went about our life as normal. I bought TV dinners for The Other to make himself to eat, because it was easy and fast, made sure I had enough cereal and milk along with a few treats. I knew I didn't want to be alone in the hospital, and we had figured that Chris's mom could stay during the day, and Chris would stay with me over night. I didn't think that was a problem since I had asked for a private room.

I had an uncle who was left alone over-night. At 11 pm, they gave him an enema and never checked on him again, by morning he was dead. His intestine perforated, and it leaked causing peritonitis—a painful way to die. I had no clue as to what they would have to do to me after surgery when I stayed there, so I knew I needed someone to be my eyes, ears, and voice.

Unfortunately, the only thing I worked on that week was making sure The Other and the house was taken care of. My girlfriend Alison was going to water my flowers every day for me. I cleaned and did the laundry, so Chris would have no worries, and I made sure I had groceries. I never once thought about what I would need after the surgery other than the couch and clean sheets on the bed. I never asked anyone who had major abdominal surgery what they did. Plus the doctor really made out like it was no big deal except for the pain, and I was ok with that.

In the days right before this major surgery, people called me from the hospital, and I went there twice, filled out more forms, and gave blood. People told me what to do the day of the surgery to prepare. Nobody ever mentioned after the surgery, and I never asked. Remember, I had set up Chris and my house, and I had clean sheets on the bed and a couch with some extra pillows and a blanket. Plus someone to water the flowers.

Major mistake on my part.

CHAPTER SEVEN
SOMEBODY HELP ME!!

I woke up the morning of the surgery very calm. I slept like I always did, on and off as I had to get up to pee that night about once an hour. I was thinking to myself that it would be nice once they got rid of the fibroid growing out of control that this peeing non-stop would finally cease. I was also hoping that the fibroid was huge and heavy so that after surgery my weight would be down. I looked forward to being able to wear all the pants that were way too tight, getting back to work, and looking sharp in some new clothes. I was hoping that when I woke up from the surgery that they would tell me that the fibroid was one of the biggest ever and that I shouldn't let going to the doctors be on the back burner. I liked this new doctor and could see me going to him yearly for check-ups; nowhere in my mind was I thinking about or preparing mentally or physically for what was to follow. Oh, I had done the obligatory research on the internet on what a fibroid was and how they removed them. I really was quite confident that in a month I would be back to work. I relied heavily that morning on the retentiveness of My Other. He had everything we needed to take assembled and ready to go, including snacks for himself. As I was worried about him sitting there and not eating, I made him eat a good breakfast and he made sure I followed the check list. The Little One (my step-son), was still at his mom's for the summer. Groceries bought, house cleaned, laundry done, grass cut, flowers tended to. Chris would get the mail on his daily trips home to shower and eat something, I really thought I had it all covered.

I was not only wrong; I was ill prepared for everything that was about to happen to me by the close of the day.

We arrived at the hospital ten minutes early. I was expecting My Other's mom and my parents to be there when I got there, but they were not. We checked in at the information desk as instructed and were handed a restaurant-style light up beeper. It went off about twenty minutes later as a woman came around the corner and called my name. The Other and I walked up to her; she took my beeper, set it on the information desk as the woman sitting at the desk highlighted my name. *"Follow me,"* she said as she walked around the corner.

We followed her to a private 6 x10 office. There was barely enough room for The Other and myself, let alone the bag of things that The Other had brought—things to entertain himself with, food to munch on; I felt horrible as I thought *I wish it was me who was waiting on someone else to have surgery*. My thoughts were interrupted by the lady who was now seated at her desk and done checking her cell phone for text messages. She asked all the usual questions you would expect: name, address, social security number, insurance, if I had a living will, medical power of attorney, and lastly, she wanted a grand upfront. I wonder to this day had I not thought to bring my credit card what she would have said to me.

From this office, she instructed us on how to get to the pre-op area: no escort, just find your way around the hospital. We did and still no parents from either side.

As we walked off the elevator, into the nice oversized waiting area, I noticed a very large flat-screen behind the reception desk with six digit numbers that were color coded. The lady placed a hospital wrist-band on me and gave The Other a card with a six digit number on it along with a name tag signifying that he was with me then she handed me a small plastic jar with a lid. It had the six digit code on it.

"Can you try and give me a sample?"

"I can pee on command, no problem," I said. Not only had I had nothing to eat or drink since 11 pm, I had already peed four times that morning–twice before leaving for the hospital and twice since I had arrived at the hospital. Just looking at a rest room sign made me want to pee.

I sat down in a chair with my sample in hand in the chair next to The Other as the parents started arriving. It seemed like an eternity in that waiting room. In actuality it was about a half an hour. Then, a man walked up to me: bald, about 6 feet tall and upwards of 250 pounds mostly situated in his stocky upper body.

Quietly he said, "Kimberly?"

"Kim," I said back and shook his extended hand. I noticed he was wearing a different color scrub then everyone else I had seen up until this point.

"You're with me Kim." He paused and looked at The Other–who's hand I didn't want to let go of. *"I will come and get you when she's all set."*

I wanted to break the ice and as we walked through the heavy doors next to the reception desk I said, *"I have some pee for you."*

He laughed and said, *"Thank you I'll add it to my collection."*

I was escorted down a long room which had a nurse's station in the center. Everyone was divided by privacy curtains; some were partially open, and I could see people laying on gurneys with loved ones gathered around holding their hands and crying. My gurney was the last one in the row. The bald guy asked the same questions the lady on the first floor did, as if to reconfirm everything he was seeing on his computer. When he asked about any allergies, I immediately spoke up on the advice of my BFF who spent several years as an ICU nurse,

"Sedatives make me nauseous."

He said he would give me something for that. Then instructed me to place everything I was wearing including all piercings and undergarments into the plastic bag that was on the gurney then put on two hospital gowns one facing forward the other facing backward and also to put on the socks that were on top of the gowns. I did as instructed. I had left all my jewelry at home, so that wasn't an issue. But, it seemed weird: tennis shoes jeans, my t-shirt and bra and underwear. I rolled everything up because the bag was clear and set the shoes on top then I got on the gurney under the thin blanket and sat up. A few minutes later, the bald guy appeared again. He gave me more pillows so I could sit more upright since lying on my back was out of the question. He had two pills for me to take for nausea, and a liquid. He said the liquid tasted bad. I laughed,

"Hey if I can do a shot of slivovitz I can do this," I drank it down like a shot. It tasted salty and rancid. He smiled. *"Wow, you can hang with the big boys!"*

"Damn straight! I have to ask." I looked him in the eye as I saw the IV paraphernalia being placed on my lap. *"How long have you been doing this?"*

"Oh, I've been a pre-op nurse for going on 18 years." Oh he's my nurse! Hence the different color scrubs.

"Just checking. I wanted to make sure that you weren't an engineer three years ago, know what I mean?"

"Oh yeah, I know. Nope, wanted to go into nursing right out of high school."

"Parents want you to be a doctor?"

"Sure enough, but the wallet said nursing school made more sense!"

He had a very relaxed way about him–like he could be one of my drinking buddies.

"Little poke," he said as he slid the needle into the top of my hand. I really didn't feel anything. I knew from experience that I wouldn't as I had watched him look at the needle to see which way the bevel was pointed.

(Here's a side note for anyone who has to have any type of needle pushed into them for any reason: tell the person doing it to make sure the needle is facing the right way. Needles have a beveled edge and when pointed correctly that little poke should be non-existent).

He explained that I would start to feel relaxed soon and to 'just go with that' feeling. Then, he said he was going to get my family and which two did I want back here with me? I asked to see Chris and my mom. I wanted Chris with me because he made me feel safe and I chose my mom over my dad because I thought her personality to be much like Chris's. Compartmentalized, strong, able to handle anything; they came through the curtain smiling. Chris came over and took my hand. We joked and talked for a while and then my mom lost it at as she decided to leave to give my dad a chance to come back. Argh! Just what I needed–crying–I found Chris's mom to be a crier at doctor's appointments. I wasn't a big crier and neither was Chris. I didn't want weeping. I needed strong people around me to keep my mind off of things. However, here was the most pulled together woman I knew, crying at my bedside. While we sat there, a nurse had come in to explain an epidural. She said the doctor recommended it for this kind of surgery. I looked at my mom who I knew had had them before when pregnant.

My mom said, *"The headache after is horrible and it makes you sick as a dog."*

The nurse said she didn't think regular pain medicine would keep me comfortable, and this might. I agreed to have one (a major mistake looking back) and signed the paper to allow the epidural, once again thinking that I had a high tolerance for pain.

After my mom left, the nurse anesthesiologist poked her head in and explained the anesthesia, how they would roll me into the operating room, and I probably wouldn't remember anything again until I woke up. She checked my teeth and asked about bridges, dentures, and partials - none of which I had.

My dad came into the curtained area for a minute or two. He was blunt and matter a fact, more like I had expected my mom to be, making statements like:

"Gosh could they make this room any smaller!"

And, *"Don't worry; one, two, three, and they'll be done."*

And, then, he was gone. My dad had recently had two separate knee surgeries, so I trusted what he said.

The actual anesthesiologist showed up next and explained the same things the nurse- anesthesiologist did. This is so they can both bill your insurance company!

My bald nurse came back in and told Chris he would have to go but to watch for my number on the large screen and it would tell them where I was in the process and that the doctor would talk to them afterwards.

Chris got up to leave as my doctor arrived. He had a brief case that was about 18 inches thick, and as he pulled out my file, I noticed he was already dressed in surgery garb, including a colorful little hat. I thought: *he looks like all the doctors I see on TV*, even sitting down once again to go over everything with me that he had discussed a week prior. He stated he would talk to my family, if that was ok with me, right after surgery, and then he would come see me in my room later on today.

He asked if I had any last minute questions, which I didn't, and then he got up walked over to the side of the gurney and took both my hands in his, he looked me right in the eye and said, *"I will do my absolute best and fix you right up!"* He smiled squeezed my hands, shook Chris's hand, picked up his files and left. Chris kissed me, said he loved me, and he would be there as soon as I woke up. I made him promise, and he did. *"Where would I go? We are the beez squared!"* and with that he also headed out past the curtains, as the bald nurse said, *"Don't worry. We'll take good care of her."*

I really didn't feel anxious or worried. I just wanted to be done. The IV was obviously working at that point because I am always over-analyzing things and that had stopped. Instead, I was paying attention to my surroundings. I had talked to a couple people who had had surgery, all of whom stated they couldn't even remember being wheeled into surgery. I knew from when they put me under during the wisdom tooth extraction that it was the best sleep I had ever had. Yet, I was trying to stay awake for some reason. I watched as they rolled me out of the curtained room. All the other curtains were pulled back now and the rooms were empty in my corridor. They whisked me past the nurses' station and then on my left out some double doors, down a short hall, and through another set of doors. It's odd to be looking at things from a laying down position. I felt like I wanted to sit up and look around. I tried hard not to look at the ceiling. When I went through the second set of double doors I realized I was in the operating room. It was much smaller than you see on TV and the ceiling was lower than I had imagined. There were two girls to my left talking about the baby that one of them had and another voice welcomed her back to work. They all seemed very happy. The equipment and lights didn't look as modern as the fictional stuff you see on TV. A voice from behind me said:

"Goodnight Kim. I will talk to you when you wake up." and with that I was out. Once again, the best sleep ever.

The next thing I heard was a loud, strong female voice.

"KIM! TIME TO GET UP! SURGERYS OVER!"

With that voice came an unbelievable pain like I had never felt before.

It was at that moment and with those words that my nightmare

really began.

As I was woken up from my surgery, the pain that was coming from my abdomen was like nothing I had ever felt. Not a stabbing pain, not an ache, more like a burning with a heavy rough brick being ground and pounded into the area.

I immediately decided that I wanted to get someone's attention, I yelled as loud as I could

"I can feel where you did the surgery! Someone help me!"

I heard a male voice *"It hurts Kim?"*

"YES IT HURTS SOMEBODY HELP ME PLEASSSSE!!!"

Now there were several voices in the back ground.

"She shouldn't have any pain."

"Maybe it's just the wear-off."

"All vitals are stable and holding."

Now I was not only in severe pain, but they were going to discuss it, I broke into their conversation:

"IT HURTS SOMEBODY HELP ME!! I NEED HELP IT HURTS SOMBODY HELP ME!!"

A woman's voice spoke up and she sternly says to me, *"Kim, remember your chart. On a scale from one to ten how much does it hurt?"*

I thought, *"Really?"* but what I said was:

"IT'S A FOURTEEN!! IT HURTS, SOMEBODY DO SOMETHING!!"

A female voice started with *"She's wide awa..."*

The voice was cut off by another voice. *"THE EPIDURAL!"*

Another voice "WHAT?"

Now, I know for sure that this pain is going to make me pass out, I felt like I was going to vomit it was so bad. I tried to yell louder and swing my arm to hit anyone I could *"SOMEBODY HELP ME!! I CAN'T TAKE THE PAIN!!!"*

Voice "THE EPIDURAL! LOG ROLL HER!"

And, at that moment, I felt my entire body being rolled over by several people lifting the sheet from my left side. I felt the blanket being removed as several hands held me on my side, a light touch on my lower back, and then as the sheet was pulled back over me I was lowered on to my back. I stopped my yelling.

"Better, Kim?" A voice came from behind me.

"Yes."

"Scale of 1-10 your pain is?" the voice asked.

"Four."

"You can tolerate it?"

"So far." The pain and the nausea had been greatly reduced with that touch I had felt on my back. I felt uncomfortable, but not overwhelmed with pain as I thought why didn't I wake up to this feeling. Idiots, forgot the epidural? I'm not really sure; I didn't ask, and I didn't care at that point.

They ran through a check sheet as people ask questions others gave answers, the whole process took less than a minute. The voice from behind me spoke again:

"We're gonna move you to a room. It might get a little bumpy. Holler if you feel an abnormal discomfort."

"Where is Chris?"

"Is Chris your husband?"

"Yes, where is he?"

"He will be up in the room."

I thought, *"Great, they don't even know who they are supposed to contact."* I didn't feel secure in the staff or what was going on around me at that moment. I remembered the lady checking her text messages when we arrived instead of doing her job. What had I gotten myself into with this hospital? As the bed I lay on started to move out of the small curtained area, we rolled through two sets of double doors and into an elevator. When the elevator doors opened we started down a hall and at some point Chris was by my side in that gurney roll about. I remember him looking anxious. They rolled me through the door of my new room, I noticed two empty beds.

"Which bed do you want Kim? Window or door?"

"I asked for a private room!"

"This is all we have, and hopefully the other bed will remain empty." They rolled and slipped me onto the bed in that same log roll fashion, I felt the bed start to move into a more upright position. There was a long narrow window next to me.

"Good luck" was what many of the voices were saying and with

that they were gone. A nice female nurse introduced herself, wrote her name on the board, and quickly went over instructions on the 'pain pump' and the 'call' button, as well as how to work the bed.

"Any questions?"

I disregarded everything she said. *"I asked for a private room."*

"I will make a note of it. We don't have any right now but if one opens up you are first on the list. Can I get you anything?"

"Not at this time."

She scurried around the room and entered information into her laptop which was on a portable stand. The aide walked in right after her and took my vitals and left. The housekeeper and another aide showed up next, bringing ice chips and asking if I needed anything. I didn't. The second Chris and I were alone he started talking, very quickly and matter-of-factly.

"The doctor came out and talked to us; you have cancer and will have to have six chemo treatments."

I couldn't believe it! I had totally talked myself out of cancer. I had done no research and read nothing about any type of cancer. I felt very behind the eight ball on information. I didn't like the feeling. I asked The Other:

"What kind of cancer and what stage. How did the surgery go? Were there any problems?"

"The surgery went well. There weren't any problems. The doctor is going to come and talk to you later on and give you all the details. I love you and I'm soooo sorry you have to go through this. Your sister Mickie is here and your mom and they want to see you."

"Ok, but first did you text Keith, Linda and Nancy?" Of course, before I had Chris notify any more family and friends I needed to let the people at work know.

"Yes, I told them you were out of surgery and doing well. I didn't tell them about the cancer. I figured you'd want to do that."

"I do. I need to process this, and have a plan. I've got to think and talk about this for a while."

I was surprised there were no tears or breakdown. I went into full Kim-the-manager mode. It's all I had to depend on at this point.

"Do you want to see your mom and sister?"

"Yes." I needed a distraction for the moment, and to ground myself.

At that moment they wheeled in a lady for the next bed. She weighted over 300 pounds, and as she was pushed through the door, she said she wanted the window. One of the staff pulled the curtain. There was the same kind of commotion as when I was brought into the room. However when she was asked if she needed anything, the woman had a laundry list of requests. This should have been my first clue to the fact that this was not going to be one of the better roommates in hospital history.

Chris left the room, briefly and soon after, my mom and my sister Michaelene walked in. Michaelene had to work that day. The drive from her work in rush hour was another forty-five minutes. I knew it had to be late in the day. I was trying to figure out how long I had been in surgery.

My sister and mom asked the usual questions of concern and we briefly discussed what I had been told. Chris came back and they left after a short visit. I requested that I have no visitors after that. I needed awhile to digest what I had been told. No longer concerned or even noticing that I was out of surgery, my mind was moving a million miles a minute, and then a nurse not dressed in scrubs, but in white lab coat walked in and sat on the edge of my bed. I had no idea why she was there or who she was or even why she thought it was ok to sit on the edge of my bed. She introduced herself by first name and said she worked on the fourth floor, but word had gotten out about my surgery and diagnosis (at that moment I had no idea what she was talking about). She took my hand and looked me in the eye and said these words:

"I want you to listen to me Kim; you get one day. One day to feel sorry for yourself and then cancer becomes your job. Don't talk to anyone for twenty-four hours. Let it sink in, and then you have to let that feeling go and make this work for you. It's the hardest thing you will ever do in your life, but I went through it twenty years ago, and they told me I wouldn't make it. And yet here I am. You can do this, but remember.... One day, that's it. Then, let it go and make it your job. OK."

She didn't ask it as a question. She spoke in low tones with no inflection. She didn't offer any other advice or emotional support. She did notice all the noise, people and activity in the bed behind the curtain, and commented right after her original statement, without giving me time to ask her any questions about what she had said to me:

"They're kinda loud," she said looking over her shoulder toward the curtain.

"Yes, it's been like this since they rolled her in." I wanted to engage this woman more. I thought maybe the doctor had sent her.

She continued the distracted train of thought, *"Let me see if I can do something about this,"* and with that she walked to the other side of the curtain. "Everyone needs to be a little quieter in here," she said to the people who had started to gather.

And with that a response from my roommate *"Can you get me some hot tea and a little something to eat?"*

"I'll send someone to help you." I heard her respond and with that she was out the door.

I looked at Chris. *"Who was that?"*

"Not sure. Maybe the doctor sent her?" (He thinks like I do.)

"Of course, I don't get to talk to her 'cause our new friend sent her on an errand."

"Why doesn't one of her family get her something?" He said loud enough so someone on the other side of the curtain would hear.

"Who knows but let's text everyone."

We then composed a text message and email to send to everyone who had asked Chris to update them, keep them posted, or mentioned they would stop by the hospital. I thought about what the mystery woman had said, and when it comes to me, she couldn't have picked better words.

My job, something I had cherished my whole life. I loved working. It made me feel in control and empowered in my life. Most importantly, until that moment, I can tell you with great certainty that my job came before everything in my life. The job was the means to everything else. In other words, it was my money. No money—no fun Kim. No money—no vacations. No money—no stuff. This woman had no idea of the impact of her words, to tell me that this *new little thing* I had going on, this cancer, needed to be my JOB.

To this day, I don't know who this woman was or why she phrased what she said like she did. I know it happened, and it wasn't a dream because My Other was sitting right next to me and heard the exact same words. Personally, I think she was an angel. Sent from God. To let me know I had a new life calling. I had never taken an illness, pain or healthcare matter seriously in my life. Definitely, nowhere near the level of priority where my job would fall.

That statement would eventually change everything about me: from the way I looked at life to how I loved, and most importantly, my own personal happiness through my tumultuous journey.

CHAPTER EIGHT
THE WORST ROOMMATE

With the mystery woman's words ringing in my ears, Chris and I started to try and settle myself into this hospital room. Chris set up the TV and phone, put the little table where I could reach it and all the things I felt I needed. Ice chips, my computer, a pen and paper, and my Aunt Jean's Red Crystal Rosary.

I was in possession of three rosaries, all of which I cherished, none of which I used with any type of regularity, one from my paternal grandmother, one from her sister, my great-Aunt Jean, and one that I got when a friend and I went to visit a weeping picture of the Virgin Mary that had traveled to a church in our area. The night before the surgery when I was putting my things together, I looked at all three rosaries, the light caught the dusty red crystals of my aunt's Rosary as they all hung from the mirror in my bedroom. My grandma had kept her rosaries hanging on the footboard of her bed, one of which was a glow-in-the dark. I knew my grandma prayed often and never missed church; it was my Aunt Jean who I watched pray the Rosary a time or two that I had spent the night at her house. She told me she watched my Uncle walk to the corner to be picked up for his ride to work, and then she would sit in the window and pray. I thought at the time that it was so peaceful sitting there looking out the window watching the traffic on the busy road go by. I wanted to start my day that way when I grow up. I never did. There was always 'something to do' or I woke up too late, or I was hung-over, and then the memory and the thought of it faded over the years. As my oldest nephew fought in Iraq, I tried several times to get into a habit of saying the prayers, but even with purpose, it never became a habit. I took my aunt's rosary and placed it with my things. It now lay in front of me on my hospital table. With all my issues and thoughts over the years of my Catholic upbringing and the 'rules' the Church puts around you, I found great comfort in that symbol lying before me.

My thoughts of the rosary and my long departed relatives were quickly halted by my doctor and surgeon coming around the closed curtain with his resident.

He stood next to the closed curtain and began to speak, with compassion and business in his voice:

"The surgery went well. We took out not just that mass we saw on the ultrasound but an additional mass behind it which was about 15 cm. We did a full hysterectomy including the cervix, omentum and an appendectomy. We got about 98% of it, the last two percent is on your diaphragm and we can't cut into that to remove it."

"What does all that mean?" I spoke remarkably calm, already half knowing the answer from what Chris had said.

"Well we are going to do six rounds of chemotherapy."

"How does that work?"

"We are going to put a port in your chest, then a week after that we will start chemotherapy. Once every four weeks, you will come back."

"When does that happen?"

"First chemotherapy should be in about three weeks."

"Can I still work?" I was panicked at the thought of not being able to work and make money.

"Oh sure. They run the cancer center all the time. We will work around your schedule, but I see no reason why you can't work."

I was beginning to feel better, and the wheels were already turning in my head. I wasn't an idiot. I knew people died from cancer all the time. I also knew many were deemed cancer free or in remission for years. I didn't know enough about this cancer, or even what kind it was. I was hoping it wasn't terminal. I continued with my next question *"Is this chemotherapy going to work. I mean what are my chances of making it through this?"*

And then it happened, the cow in the next bed had been vying for attention since the moment she came in the room. If she didn't have a visitor or someone to talk to, she would throw a pen at the doorway when a person would walk by and ask them to pick it up for her, when they returned the pen she would try to start a conversation. This irritant was compounded by the fact that on one of Chris's trips out of the room to get my mom and sister, her visitors came around the curtain and tried to take the chair out of my side of the room, which would leave nothing for Chris to sit on. I was furious when the pen hit my doctor's foot as I asked the question about my chances for survival.

Now, most people have seen the inside of a hospital room, and the curtain that divides the beds, my doctor spoke in a calm voice, but he was by no means a quite talker, and there is no way that this woman could not have heard the conversation.

The doctor looked down at the pen, and the voice came from behind the curtain *"Oops I dropped my pen again. Excuse me can you please hand me my pen?"*

The doctor ignored her as did the resident, and with the *"excuse me, excuse me, can you..."* fading into background and turned into white noise. The doctor continued:

"80/20." He said with great confidence. *"This treatment works in about 80% of the people and will eliminate the rest of the cancer."*

"What if it doesn't work?" I asked

"We'll deal with that when and if we get to it," he again said most confidently.

"Ok, so what kind of cancer is this?" I asked again wanting confirmation of what I had already been told.

"We won't know for sure till the lab tests come back, but I am reasonably sure that we are looking at Ovarian Stage III."

My anxiety level rose at the word. Not Ovarian... but *Stage III*. I knew there were four stages in cancer and I was mortified that I was in stage three! I listened as the doctor explained the staging and why mine was considered three. I kept thinking: how the hell did this happen, Stage three? I began to worry, never really thinking about the word Ovarian, just the words Cancer and Stage three.

The doctor finished his staging explanation and started to explain the office procedures to start the process. He ended his statement with, *"Kim do you have any more questions? I will stay as long as you need to answer them."*

"Umm, I'm good right now. I'm sure some will come up later on."

"Call the office anytime with any questions. All of my oncology nurses

can help you or they can find me to ask the question."

"Ok, I want a private room. I asked for one, and they didn't give me one." I said glancing towards the curtain of the patient in the next bed still talking out-loud to no one and everyone.

The doctor looked at the resident, and she looked at me,

"We're working on it. You are next on the list."

He grabbed my hands in his again, *"It's a privilege and an honor,"* and with that he left with his resident. The other side of the curtain now had an aide in it answering the cries of "excuse me my pen."

I looked at My Other,

"Well eighty percent is pretty good."

"We can do this!" And with his smile I knew I could and everything would work out. I just knew.

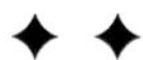

Later in the evening, I was assigned a male nurse. He was pleasant, wrote his name on the board, and took my vitals. He, like the other girl, asked questions about how I was feeling. I couldn't really say at that point. Chris sat next to me in the chair holding my hand. We started to plan. It is what we do best—get it straight in our heads how it is all going to work. Our ingenious plan was to get me home in a day or two, schedule the port insertion for exactly two and a half weeks from the date of surgery with chemotherapy a week later. I wrote on a piece of paper the dates on Fridays. It worked out perfectly. I could have two chemo's down before they even expected me back at work. I would take four Fridays off unpaid, recover on the weekends, and be done with this before the end of the year. It all made sense. Chris sat with me as the hours passed and it became dark outside the windows. I was looking at this as something I could put parameters around. Manage and control like almost every aspect of my life. I would control the cancer and the treatment of it. **insert insane laughter here**

Chris thought he could doze off in the uncomfortable upright chair. The visitors of my roommate had stopped, but she didn't shut down. She was still throwing her pen. Her guests had brought her a large paper grocery bags full of junk food, and the constant rustling of plastic chip bags and cookie wrappers was magnified by the silence of the hospital. Visiting hours had been over for awhile and at 11pm the male nurse came in and said Chris had to leave. He was a male in a woman's room after visiting hours. I was devastated. I knew that would happen without a private room and immediately regretted not having my mom or Chris's mom stay. He left and I was alone. Without the distraction of another person I noticed how uncomfortable I really was. I had no one to help me move. I was a side sleeper so even being propped up sleep was not coming.

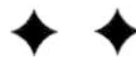

I had had an irregular heartbeat earlier in the day. It was something that had been happening on occasion since I was a child, maybe once or twice a year, but since I was in the hospital when it happened I asked for the nurse to check my heart. She ordered what they call the RAT team to come up. They were there in thirty seconds and had me hooked up to a monitor. The doctors quickly diagnosed the issue. Nothing for me to be concerned with. However, The Rapid Response Team had ordered blood drawn every four hours. Even though they never turned on a light, they would wake me to draw if I was dozing, in addition to taking vitals every couple hours. The call speaker next to the bed went off every half hour or so telling the nurse or aides which room they were needed in. Then there was the roommate. She had to be helped to the bathroom several times from all the soda-pop and goodies she was eating. At midnight, she was hooked to a breathing machine which sounded like loud snoring to me. Sleep did not come at all the first night. I tried to watch TV but the stations were limited and the ones they did get were showing infomercials. I couldn't read. I couldn't write. I had nobody to talk to for hours and hours. I could only lay there feeling sick to my stomach and worry. I held on to the rosary my great-aunt Jean had given me hoping it would bring me some kind of comfort and watched the minutes on my phone click off slowly. It was eight hours until Chris could come back at 7am. It felt like days. By the time morning came I was so incredibly angry about the lack of sleep because of my roommate and the interruptions plus the fact that no one could stay with me; I waited for the day nurse. She was the same girl from yesterday. She asked me how I slept. I told her I didn't and in a low voice explained about the roommate and the eating and calling the aides all night. I don't mind the hospital workers having to do their job, but that's an unnecessary annoyance with the constant voice over the speaker.

I had said that the surgery was the best sleep of my life. Yet it was only four or five hours, and considering the lack of sleep leading up to the surgery, I was now exhausted from an entire night of not even being able to sleep for a few hours. The nurse said they had a private room coming; they were just waiting for the person to be released.

I could see the sympathy in the day nurses eyes. She had been with me for less than five minutes and my roommate had already asked her for hot tea and to be moved to a chair. She patiently explained she would be with her next, but the interruptions kept coming.

Ovarian Cancer is not one of fashionable cancers; there is not a lot of money being spent on its research. Except for Gilda's House, which are sporadic around the country, there is no large organization spreading the word about the silent symptoms. Yet, it is the DEADLIEST OF THE GYNECOLOGICAL CANCERS.

In 2011 there were just under 22,000 new cases of ovarian cancer. That same year, 15,000+ women didn't survive ovarian cancer.

CHAPTER NINE

THE FUN BEGINS *INSERT SARCASM HERE*

By the end of day two I had been moved into one of the few isolation rooms on the floor. I started to get more comfortable with my surrounding in that isolation room. In the double room, I had spent the day trying to talk to the resident who came to see me in the morning and the nurses to try and compile information on how to recover from this surgery quickly. (Remember I thought I'd be going home in three to four days.) I couldn't speak with anyone in the first room because of the interruptions. In the private room I could hear myself think once again. I noticed for the first time since I could remember that I didn't have to pee, and the thought crossed my mind about having to get up and go to the bathroom. Although I knew I was going on 40 hours with no food or real beverages, I couldn't figure out why I didn't have to go. Until the aide showed up to empty the plastic pitcher attached to my catheter.

"Oh baby," the middle aged woman said as she held the pitcher in the air noticing only a few ounces of a dark yellowish-brown heavy liquid. *"You've got to be drinking yourself a lot more! This should be full and light yellow."*

"What is that?" I said half knowing.

"It's your pee from your catheter baby. You've got to start drinking more."

Up until that moment, I had no idea that I had a catheter in. It was strange. I always thought one would hurt but I felt nothing at all. I lost the fear of having to get up to go to the bathroom which meant I could now ask the question I didn't want to ask, *"What can I have?"*

The aide looked at my board on the wall and pointed to the bottom corner. *"See clear liquids."*

I realized that someone had written that on the board at some point, however I hadn't noticed it.

"What does that mean?" I asked her.

"Ice, water, sprite, broth, popsicles, gelatin, let me bring you something," she said as she looked into the pitcher of half-melted ice chips I had been slowly chomping on all night.

"Ok." I was so happy. *"Ice water and a popsicle!"* I loved popsicles as a kid and was happy to be getting one and some cold water to drink.

I continued to drink water with the nudging reminders of My Other's mom. By the next pee cup change, the container was half-full and bright yellow.

"Oh good job baby! Keep it up!"

The second day passed into evening. The Other and his mom worked out a schedule per my request, so one of them could always be there. We double checked with the nurse about Chris staying at night with me in this room and she agreed.

I slept on and off that night while I watched Chris try to sleep between two chairs. I knew he was uncomfortable; however, I felt so much better knowing he was there.

As I entered my third day, the headache and upset stomach started. The doctor ordered the epidural removed. Up until that point, I had been given a series of pills every few hours; stool softeners, pain killers, antibiotics, and medicines for the nausea. I took all of them without question but texted and called Charlotte over and over for anything I didn't know or understand.

Once the epidural was out, a few hours later the nurses wanted me to work on sitting up in a chair. With assistance from the nurse I was able to get into a chair. My legs still wobbled from the epidural. Sue helped me change hospital gowns, clean up and get ready to received visitors in my chair. It was like holding court; friends and family came and went for about two hours, all well-choreographed by Chris to run at my convenience not the schedules of those who wanted to come. Do not be afraid to speak up to family and friends and say to them: *'you can come at this time only.'* Also, as a patient, please understand that many people can't stomach hospitals. Don't be offended for those who can't make it or they can't come because of scheduling issues; it doesn't mean they don't love or care about you. In addition, family and friends who are visiting, leave your opinions and issues at the door. Nobody who is lying in a hospital bed recently diagnosed with cancer wants to listen to you about your problem teenager or irritating coworker. I was lucky. My friends and family came in full throttle to make me laugh, and they succeeded in taking my mind off my troubles for a few hours. My friend Keith was the biggest instigator and used my love of vodka to get worried looks out of the aide every time he walked in the room. I am sure that aide and his numerous visits in a two hour period where to make sure Keith wasn't feeding me vodka. Even though as he did remark within earshot of the aide, *"vodka is a clear liquid and therefore should be on the list of things I could consume."*

The remainder of the day passed without much incident. The catheter was removed and Chris and his mom helped me start to walk from the bed to the bathroom. I couldn't do it on my own yet, but I was peeing by myself and I thought that was a good sign. Night came and it was another restless one for both Chris and me. He couldn't get comfortable on the chairs, and I was in full insomniac mode, trying to keep quite watching TV. At 4 am, I had Chris help me to the bathroom and when he got me back into bed I said to him:

"Why don't you head home and get some real sleep. Your mom will be here in three hours. I won't drink anything so I won't have to get up before she gets here."

"Are you sure?" He said with some question. But I knew him, if he didn't get some real sleep soon he was going to lose it.

"Yes, I've been fine all day. I will be ok. Go, and I want you to shut off your phone so no one bother you and set your alarm for 1 pm so you get a full 8 hours. You need it. Go your mom will be here at seven."

He jumped at the chance to leave and get some real sleep but worried about leaving me. I kept reassuring him and he left.

That was a mistake on my part. I knew I needed someone with me 24-7. I KNEW that. Still, I put Chris's well-being in front of my own. Qualifying it with, it's only three hours. What can happen in three hours?

At 5 am, the night nurse had come in to check my vitals, and I must say someone was watching out for me. As she chatted like she did the night before about her sister who has breast cancer, I started to feel nauseous. I told the woman I thought I was going to throw up, and she handed me a four by six inch dish that was about two inches deep. I held it under my mouth and a watery like substance came up. She took the dish from me, rinsed it and gave it back to me and left the room. *What the hell*, I thought, I was ready to heave again and I held it back with all I had, remembering the heavy nights of drinking in my late teens and early twenties, head spinning, foot over the edge of the bed trying desperately not to heave.

I reached for my phone and dialed Chris - right to voice mail, damn-it. He followed my instructions. I left a voice mail just in case, and called Chris's mom. Voice mail. I knew it was futile. I only had two hours to go. I left her a message to come early if she could.

The aide checked on me. He was in his 30's and reminded me of the ER nurse I had. He showed up for the night shift happy and telling me the Tigers scores and his opinion of the pitching. I told him I was going to be sick. He got me a larger container and set a second container on the chair next to the bed. Ok, I was good with that for a couple of hours, I asked him for the popular name brand ginger ale. We called it 'medicine pop' around our house, his family did also. He tried to joke about it.

To try and calm my stomach I tried sipping it, but whatever I sipped, it came back up. Chris's mom showed up at 7:30 and the real fun began. My stomach began churning, and the diarrhea started. Now Sue was trying to get me to the bathroom in time for me to sit there and vomit in a bucket. Both ends, this was not pleasant. The doctors put me on ice chips again. I would fill my mouth with ice, try to crush it up more with my teeth, and then spit it out right before I vomited. This seems weird. However, you start to vomit all the medicines that have been in your body since the day of the surgery. My vomit was neon green at one point, the ice would cool off the inside of my mouth and ease some of the burning caused by what was coming out. The diarrhea started out as mostly water. Annoying, mildly painful, but tolerable…at first.

In the final hours of day four the worst started to hit me. I had been complaining all day of being sick to my stomach. They tried a few different anti-nausea medications, none of which seemed to be working. The male night aide had checked in a few times, sneaking me pop and ice that I promised him I wouldn't swallow just spit out as I vomited. I had been regulated on the second half of the day to a wet sponge around the mouth. It didn't matter. Everything I put in my mouth tasted strange anyways. My taste-buds seemed to be a little off. The pop, the sugary popsicles, all had shifted in taste in a matter of hours and although I had not ingested anything, there were still flavors going into my mouth that I should have been able to taste; I likened it to the constant vomiting. I woke Chris up from his chair.

"I have to get to the bathroom."

"Ok, I'm coming." And before he could stand up to help me, I could feel my insides release, and this time it was different than the water that had been coming out. He helped me hobble to the bathroom dragging the ever present IV pole with me. I left a trail of crap from the bed all the way to the bathroom. I could feel it running down both of my legs as I made it to the toilet and Chris shut the door. I could hear him say as I vomited all over myself:

"Don't worry, I'll get this cleaned up."

And I started to cry for the first time. I was covered in shit and vomit. It was going on five days that I hadn't showered or washed my hair. My stomach and lower back were now violently cramping with each morsel that exited my body. My head was pounding from the never ending headache they had determined was caused by the epidural. I hadn't eaten anything for days or drank anything in hours. The cancer was the farthest thing from my mind. What I wanted to know was when this was going to stop and when I could get the hell out of this place!

I realized how totally unprepared I was for all of this. Nobody, not once said any of this was going to happen. That I would vomit and have violent unexpected diarrhea, that my head would hurt, or I wouldn't be able to eat or drink. I would have prepared myself differently. I was upset and angry at everyone and everything. How the hell was I going to clean myself off? I had shit all up and down both legs! There were no towels in this bathroom I could even get wet to try.

I heard noises and talking outside my door. Chris had gotten the aide. He was changing the bed and had the janitor come mop the floor. I got up and peeked out:

"Can I get a couple on new hospital gowns and some washcloths and a towel?" I asked the aide.

"Housekeeping left you a bunch of stuff here." He pointed to the top of the sink, *"These ones are wrecked though."* As he tossed some rolled up blankets into a bag, I realized that housekeeping had been leaving me towels and gowns rolled up tight in these packages. I had used them, thinking they were rolled up blankets to prop myself into comfortable sleeping positions. My thought was broken with the male aide's voice.

"I'm going to get my partner on the floor to come help you clean up. She'll be right here." With that he picked up the bag of crap covered sheets and blankets and headed out the door. A few moments later, I heard a knock on the bathroom door

"Kim, can I come in?" I heard a quite female voice.

"Yeah." I said half-heartedly.

She closed the door behind her and said, *"Can you stand for a few moments for me?"*

"I'm afraid I'm going to go to that bathroom all over you if I stand to long," I said with tears in my eyes.

She started laughing. *"Well, you wouldn't be the first to do that, but don't worry you should be fine now. That was the big release after a surgery like yours."*

"What?" I was surprised by the comment, and stood up.

"I got these from the heater. They are warm, so this should feel good." She ignored my "What?" in reference to the 'big release' statement as she wiped down both legs. It was humiliating to have a stranger have to do this; in fact it would have been humiliating no matter who had to do this to me. She was happy and polite and chatted about her children–making small talk to make me feel better. She asked if I wanted her to wipe off my butt or should she? How polite of her. How horribly embarrassing for me, especially when I had to have her do it. I had IVs in the top of both hands and couldn't do a good job myself.

I slowly walked on my own, clutching the IV pole and asked the aide to bring some diapers back. So this is what I am reduced to I thought. My aide returned with some heavy pads, he told me to place them on the bed under me.

"Can I get some diapers?"

"I'll bring some. You can put them under you."

"Are they too hard to get on?" I asked not knowing what the big deal was. I had watched and helped my parents with all four of my grandparents. I knew the routine with adult diapers. It sucked, but I felt it was necessary at this point.

"You can't cover up your scar just yet." He set the pads down on the sink and left.

I wanted to look at my surgery cut now. Up until this point the resident and nurses had checked it. I had only let Sue look at it. They told me no more bandages about 16 hours after surgery. Each time the resident checked it she would say that it was doing remarkable. The nurses also had been commenting about how well and quickly it was healing. I hadn't looked at it up until this point. Chris had settled back in his chair and I pulled up my gown. I was shocked… I grew up the last years of the baby boomers generation. Born in 1962, we were the last year of the generation, old enough to be lumped in, but young enough to enjoy all the modern miracles that have come to pass over the last 30 years, one of them being surgeries. I knew so many people who, after surgery, would show off this tiny little scar. I always thought it was amazing how much they could do with lasers and scopes, not really creating much of a scar or too many problems in healing. Then, there are those of us who don't concentrate on what is really going on, and when a doctor says, 'We are going to take out all the goodies' and you say to him 'Ok but take everything it is touching' that is the go ahead for 'exploratory surgery'. Did I need that? Absolutely! Was I prepared for that? Absolutely Not!

My incision started about two inches above my belly button and continued down until about an inch under my pubic area. It was incredibly long and very unexpected on my part. I saw the silver staples and was kind of irritated that they weren't the dissolvable type, so I wouldn't have to go through the hassle of making another appointment to get the staples out. This is where my mind always went…How soon will it be before I can get back to the place where I go to work every day and don't have to take time off for doctor. I was less than a week into this, and I was thinking exit strategy.

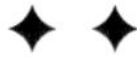

All day Sunday the experience of getting to crap myself happened over and over, I got more used to the warning signs, and as my bowels emptied out the heavy brown mess turned back to brown water. The doctors wanted me up and walking… I thought to myself, I am walking, back and forth to the bathroom every fifteen minutes.

Monday morning arrived, I knew I had had nothing to eat since last Tuesday night, and with the removal of the two large masses I thought I needed a boost to my moral. I want to walk to a scale and weigh myself. Sue and I ventured into the hall a few steps to weigh in. I had gained twelve pounds. Not really the boost I was looking for. It never occurred to me to ask why there was a weight gain. I thought to myself: *"just my luck, the only person ever to not eat for a full week after a major surgery and still gain weight!"*

I was relieved when the resident on her morning stop-in said I could go home that evening. I was also a little shocked. I still could barely walk from one room to another. The diarrhea hadn't stopped completely. I was getting used to it and able to control it a bit more. The vomiting had stopped and the headaches. The nurse came in after the resident's visit and said I need to eat a meal by tonight and I could leave. I ordered food from the restricted menu for lunch and dinner, neither of which tasted right.

My dad was visiting and he said just eat it. He picked up the hamburger took a bite and said, "It's not that bad." Then fifteen minutes later told the nurse the food wasn't edible! I made Chris go get me a fast food hamburger and fries. It didn't taste like it should, and by the time I got it, the fries were cold. I pitched all the food and told the nurse I ate the hamburger and drank a chocolate shake. At 9 pm on Monday evening, they released me from the hospital.

What a stupid thing. I should have insisted on staying that night and going home in the morning.

When we pulled up in the driveway of our home, the neighbor across the street was out on her porch smoking. She came running across the street volunteering to help get me in the house. Since Chris had already opened the door, and I was walking slowly with his assistance, I took the translation in that comment to be *"What is going on, me and the neighbors want to know so I'll help you and hopefully you will tell me."* Chris and I think exactly alike in certain situations and nosy neighbors who smell like cigarettes is one of them.

"We got this thanks," was his sharp reply back to her. *"Translation, Go back to your cigarettes. This is none of your business."*

I walked in the door and felt such a sense of relief and comfort. It no longer smelled like antiseptic soap and vomit... I could smell my vanilla candles. As I slowly made it around the corner to the bathroom the ferry flower oil I loved so much wafted from the tiny space. I bought the specialty oils and soaps from a local woman who makes them herself. And the smell of them soothed my every fiber. I removed the diaper I had adorned myself with for the ride home and put on some clean pajamas. I felt better being in my own clothing.

We had stopped at the closest fast food place so I could get some hot French fries, and I sat on the couch and ate one. It tasted bland, but I ate another one and a grain of salt got stuck in my throat. I started to cough. Terrified that I would rip my stitches, I firmly grabbed a pillow put it over my surgery incision and started to yell. I wanted pop or water to wash it out and stop the coughing. I couldn't cough and expressed the urgency that I needed something to drink. I yelled more and louder as I watched Chris and thought he wasn't moving fast enough.

Scared to death! We fought, something we had NEVER done in our ten plus years together.

That's right, Chris and I had been together for all those years, in blissful happiness, the wedding we planned was only icing on the cake for us. We had gone all this time and never even raised our voices to each other, let alone fight about things like getting a drink. If something bothered one or the other, we spoke up and talked and resolved it right then and there, never letting things linger and definitely never yelling at each other over something as petty as the speed at which one was getting a drink. After the verbal barrage, I started to cry for a second time in as many days. He sat down next to me. We agreed that I would be specific about what I needed and he would let me know what he was doing instead of leaving me hanging.

✦ ✦

We knew we needed to get settled in and get me to sleep. Every thought and assumption that Chris and I made to 'prepare' me for post-surgery was incorrect.

Chris went into our room, the shortest walk to the bathroom, and a straight line at that. He took stiffer pillows from our couch and placed our regular pillows on top creating that half upright position that had worked in the hospital. Our bed is on risers. We did this because we are both tall and liked the look. Because we lived in a post-WWII bungalow and had little storage space, the extra room under the raised bed left us with an area to store plastic boxes full of out-of-season or seldom-used items. Only today, I stood there trying to figure out how I was going to get up there. Chris grabbed the step I used to reach high shelves; I stood on the small step, turned around, and gently sat down on the bed. OK, that works, he helped me lay back. At last in my own bed! I flipped on the TV to watch a show I liked instead of the crap they showed in the hospital. We kept laughing at the adult cartoon rerun, and I joked to stop making me laugh before I ripped my staples out. All was alright, for about a half hour more, then I had to go to the bathroom. Chris had put old towels and some of those pads from the hospital under me so I wasn't concerned about making a mess, but I realized at that moment, in the hospital, the bed had railings on either side about a quarter of the way down the bed, and I had been using my arms to pull myself up by grabbing onto the railings. I had nothing to grab onto, and no way to sit up to swing my legs over the bed. I woke up the now dozing off Chris.

"I can't sit up."

"Let me help you." He sat up and turned to try and lift me.

"No give me your arm."

He held out his arm straight. I grabbed it and pulled myself up. Upon my return, it was harder to get into the bed without Chris holding me. I had to get up again about a half an hour later. This time I tried to push myself up off the nightstand. It didn't work and I had to wake Chris out of a solid sleep. I was exhausted and frustrated.

"I can't sleep in the bed."

"Ok, let's try the couch," he said through his grogginess.

He had set the couch up for what we thought would be me sitting there working from home. Covered in a blanket and then a sheet, our two-piece, hand-me-down was pushed together in the usual L-shape. I sat on one side. It had a sofa sleeper in it and sank really low. The other side wasn't that much better. The couch had three individual cushions on each side and I would fall in between those cushions. Chris tried blankets, pillows. Nothing seemed to work to firm up the cushions and keep them still. It was going on 2am and we still hadn't slept. I wished now I was still back in the hospital in the hospital bed.

"I am not the only person in the world to have this surgery! How the hell do people do this?!"

"They have recliners," he snapped back even more irritated.

That made sense. Of course we didn't own a recliner. However, if we would have thought about it in advance, or someone would have said something, we could have bought or borrowed one. Chris kept going from room to room looking for the right pillow or item that would work. Then I saw him emerge from the basement with the doors from a freestanding closet. He put one under each section and then on top of the cushion separation he placed a pillow from off the bed and wrapped the couch tight in a blanket. He used the rest of the pillows to make an upright seat. All this took another hour and then we realized we needed to actually separate the couches, so I could use the larger arm rest from the corner section. By 3:30 in the morning we were settled, with me on the newly jury-rigged couch with a backwards folding chair next to me to grab and be able to hoist myself up. A small table now set up with pills, water and the TV remote, only I was facing backwards from where the TV was. Our living room was destroyed with furniture pushed aside and out of the way. Part of our couch was randomly in the middle of the room and I lay there pissed at myself for not being prepared, thinking about all the things I should have done.

The questions I should have asked and wondering why nobody said anything. They asked me several times in the hospital from the check-in to the check-out, how many stairs were in my house, but nobody ever asked about how I was going to sleep or sit in my own house. I also started worrying about our bathroom. Our very small home came with one very small bathroom, and I had no control over when I was going to go. How was Chris going to be able to use the bathroom?

It was all starting to be too much for me. Too much for me… ME! There was no one in my life more organized and prepared for anything and everything. Second only to me was Chris, yet we were so far behind the eight-ball on being prepared post-surgery at home.

CHAPTER TEN

THE FIRST OF SEVERAL PROBLEMS ARISE

The hours turned into days and as I became more aware of the daytime TV schedule, and might I add if anyone high enough in TV programming ever gets to this book, contact me and I will let you know what people who watch the programs all day actually think of your idiotic programming. But I digress, the irritant of the lack of something to take my mind off my misery was such a small thing compared to the physicality of what was happening to my body. The realization of instant menopause had set in. One second I was shivering cold and the next I was sweating uncontrollably. I remember the little segment they did on a morning news show when some woman tried to show the male host of the show what a hot flash was–I laugh to think she wasn't even close. The woman placed an electric blanket on high and piled a bunch of blankets on him as he lay on a couch. Piece of cake I say! You are just laying there! You need to actually function during a hot-flash and the feeling of being over heated is nothing. The heat you experience clings to your skin so even if you remove your clothes your body radiates a moist heat that you can't wipe off like you would normal perspiration.

If you want to know what a hot flash feels like, I can help you simulate one. Now this works best in a colder month of the year or you can turn your air-conditioning down to a setting about 10 degrees colder than you are used to. First, dress head to toe in an itchy or rough wool outfit: including wool socks and a wool hat and wrap your neck with a wool scarf and place wool gloves on your hands (no cotton or soft underwear-those parts sweat too!). Now, go into your bathroom and shut the door. Put a towel at the base of the door where it meets the floor. Turn your shower on HOT water only and point the shower head against the wall so it starts to spray and steam. Make sure you are sitting (outside the tub-not in the scalding water)… and wait. You will see the bathroom start to fill with steam: don't turn on your fan or open a window and don't remove any clothing. You will start to feel the sweat: your head, your neck; it will run down the middle of your back to your butt. Your feet and fingers will start to sweat. Don't wipe it off (you can't wipe this feeling off during a hot flash) Stay in that room after the sweating begins for at least 2 full minutes (no matter how bad it gets, remember your girlfriend, wife, sister, mom can't leave). After two minutes, leave the bathroom and as fast as you can strip down to your underwear and either stand in front of your most powerful air-conditioning vent or step outside in the cool winter air. Don't wipe that sweat off you. Feel the stickiness turn to cold, clammy irritability. That's what a hot-flash feels like. Oh and those soaking wet clothes you left behind, that's what your pajamas feel like after a night sweat occurs. Think about what you went through: did you make it? Or did you tear off your clothing early? Did you wipe up the sweat because it bothered you? Did you have to remove your gloves because it felt like your hands were suffocating?

I want you to also keep in mind that is *one* of the menopausal side-effects. There is the uncontrollable irritability. Not knowing it, but the uncontrollable anger that lead to my and Chris's into a fight was the first time I experienced it. I found myself angry for no particular reason. I would awake from a nap and be in a bad mood and that was something that I had never gone through before. I thought I was speaking in my usual tones and with my regular 'Kim' attitude. I found out on the other side of surgery recovery that I was speaking like an ass to My Other and The Little One. They both hid it from me until they felt they could confront me with it.

After that conversation, I made a choice in my life that when I woke up in a bad mood I would first tell them straight up, "I woke up angry." They would both go out of their way to be very nice to try and dispel the mood, and I would literally confront every thought I had when it came to my emotions. If I was driving and became irritated with someone, I would think: *"Do I need to be angry? Did someone physically do something to me?"* I continued that train of thought throughout the day, questioning every upset, angry, or irritated emotion. Which also lead to me analyzing every emotion.

As a teenager going through puberty, I cried a lot. We had four girls in our house. Someone was always crying. Once I made it through those years, I bottled up many of those crying jaunts. I worked for thirteen years in a place where the owners made the female personnel feel like garbage on a very regular basis. At least once a week there was a female employee in the ladies room balling her eyes out and venting to me. When I took the hit I refused to let them push me to that point. I would call a friend or My Other for moral support and ask the question *"Why shouldn't I tell these people to piss off?"* Each one would take a minute with me explaining why I needed my job. I would turn my emotions to anger, never letting anyone see me cry. Now I found myself getting choked up at movies and TV commercials. Things that would happen during the day, and eventually chemotherapy would bring me to tears. The crying fits were met with confusion by My Other, having never had to deal with me crying or in any type of highly charged emotional state. His statement to my tears was at first,

"Do you need to go to the emergency room?"

Which of course would make me angry and I would think to myself, *"yeah, they will give me that new pill which stops people from crying or being emotional"*.

These new found menopausal side-effects were much more intense than the things I was going through pre-surgery - thinking I was in menopause. However, they were a piece of cake compared to the post-surgery side-effects. The big one, the one that everyone keeps silent about; it not only happens to people who have hysterectomies and exploratory surgery, it happens to anyone who has their abdominal region opened up.

Your bowels coming back to normal.

Here is the dirty little secret that nobody tells you about. And even though you are going to think it can't get much worse than what I am about to tell you, I would remind you that it is going to. I would also like to add if this alone doesn't force you into a doctor's office yearly, then, like me, you run that risk of getting to experience this yourself.

When in the hospital I asked the resident each morning when she arrived about my surgery, what was happening to me as I got sicker and what else was headed my way. Her answer was always the same:

"Well, everybody's different, and when you have an invasive surgery where the bowels are touched, examined, or like in my case, removed from my body and set on a table while they checked the rest of me, they go into shock and have to re-start themselves."

I thought that meant that the liquids that were pouring out of my ass were the restart of my bowels. Yeah… no such luck. Those liquids as I mentioned where primarily the fluids that they pump into you via IV. No your bowels actually have to 'retrain' themselves to pass a more solid mass.

Bowels run into the colon, which creates contractions or waves to push the stool into the rectum and out of the body. Restarting this process is painful beyond anything you can imagine. Women who have had C-sections sometime experience this pain if their bowels have been touched. It doesn't matter if you take a stool softener or a laxative. In fact, I found the use of these things actually slowed down the restart process. There is nothing you can do except tough it out.

As your bowels and colon start to begin the processes of forming a more solid stool and moving it down, it starts to cramp. Ever wonder why some babies cry when they have to poop, it hurts. The pain of the contraction restarting and the movement in to the rectum cause a pain that will make you have to hold on to something: the edge of the sink, the window sill, the tub. I brought a folding chair into the bathroom so I could hang onto the back of it. If you were to hold onto say a full roll of toilet paper it will make you shred through that roll with your fingers. To simulate the pain, I would say that while you are having stomach pains caused by diarrhea, from say eating spoiled food, have someone punch you in the stomach. And then if you are a man, have someone kick you in the balls on top of it or for a women, think about your worse period cramps combined with diarrhea cramping and contractions in childbirth. It is a pain so intense it will make you scream out loud with relief when you finally pass a stool. But the fun isn't over because once you pass it, there will be more behind it that will sit there until several hours later. I longed to have the 'crap myself' phase back in lieu of this new phase of going to the bathroom. That pain started about ten days after my surgery and lasted for about seven days. Building up and getting more intense and then tapering off at the end and turning back into diarrhea before it eventually regulated to my normal once a day bowel movement.

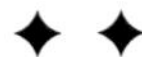

With the addition of the bowel restart on top of all the new menopause symptoms plus the fact that I had had major surgery and I would be laying in one spot all day and all night long, my normally highly charged and active life style had come to a screeching halt. By that, I mean physically. I had gone from a full-time job, taking care of our home, exercising regularly, plus the part-time work of housecleaning and helping with the band, to walking the fifteen feet or so back and forth to the bathroom three dozen times a day. It was a shock to the system. Chris tried to encourage me to get up off the couch and walk but it was painful and embarrassing to do so. I was able to work two weeks after surgery but that only entailed me sitting on the couch and using my laptop. No heavy lifting or any type of exercise. I was thankful for the distraction but it didn't help me physically. I thought by the third week I would be able to move around a bit more; however that wasn't meant to be...

A few days after I arrived home I also made a call as directed to the doctor's office to set up the port insertion, staple removal and the start of chemotherapy. The doctor had been very plain and very understandable when he said,

"Chemo will start in three weeks. One week after we install a port."

I was surprised and irritated when I called to schedule and an oncology nurse had to phone me back. It took another phone call to the office and more than twenty-four hours after that second call to get a call back only to hear:

"I've scheduled you for stitches to be removed next Wednesday, a meeting the day before your port surgery with a nurse and then the surgery." In what would have been 6 weeks from the major surgery, then chemo ten days after that. Seven and a half weeks.

I thought to myself: "*That doesn't work.*" I wanted two chemos out of the way before I went back to work, plus the doctor had said *I would be starting chemo in about three weeks.* I felt a sense of urgency as I didn't want to have the cancer spread anywhere beyond the diaphragm. The time she was stating was more than double what the doctor had said. Also, I was a bit put off that nobody asked what days were good for me. After all I had to provide my own rides along with people to take care of me and that meant scheduling around other peoples' lives.

I choose to go with what the doctor said,

"Umm, the doctor said port surgery and then chemo at three weeks. I was thinking July 23rd for the port insertion and July 30th for first chemo."

"That's too soon!" she practically screamed into the phone.

"That's what the DOCTOR told me!" I responded, trying not to get upset as I felt the tears already starting to well up.

"Listen, I've been doing this for twenty-three years, and you can't have that first chemo before four weeks."

She quickly retorted, *"And there is the surgery, and meeting before the surgery and your stitches need to be removed."*

"Check with the doctor! Don't you have my chart or something with his notes!" I knew my voice was starting to get shrill but not getting in two chemo's before I had to be back at work was not in my plan.

"Listen I'm NOT going to schedule you that quick," she argued.

"Check with the doctor!" I said now in full blown tears as I hung up the phone.

Like I said, it took two calls and a decent waiting period before they called me back the first time. I could only imagine how long this was going to take. I waited until I calmed down and called the office back. I tried not to get irritated as I spoke with the original girl who fit me in. I explained what happened with the nurse. She was incredible understanding and said she would see what the problem was and have someone call me back shortly. The phone rang an hour later. It was the same nurse with a gentler disposition.

"Ok Kim, I spoke with the doctor and we have your dates lined up."

"Ok, I've got a pen."

She proceeded to tell me dates which made my port surgery the last week in July and the first chemo on August 13. She also told me about the three blood draws I would need to go for and the consultations as well as the staple removals. All in all, in about a four week period. I would have to be driven back and forth to the hospital six times, each requiring the help of someone as I was not ready to walk yet any type of distance.

I didn't argue with the nurse as the dates were closer to what the doctor said and at that point I just wanted to get it scheduled. I had always hated calling any type of office to schedule anything. You can never get the date and time you want unless you call six months in advance, and even then it was iffy. Forget an after work or weekend appointment also. Cancer, in my case, was going to have to fall into 'banker's hours' which severely limited who could take me to my appointments. I knew from the start that that would be a problem. I was starting to see a pattern of continuous appointments, and asking people to take time off work was not going to be fair to anyone close to me.

I put a lot of time and thought into who I wanted to accompany me on all these outings. My first choice of course was my Other or my Mom. My Other had to work to support us and my mom had to take care of my ailing dad. My best friend had a job that she traveled for and a new baby who was born prematurely. All fingers were pointing to one person: My Other's mom. She was the most logical choice. Retired, available, and sympathetic to my illness, I knew however that she was already stretched taking care of other people. While I was contemplating all of this, I received an email from my friend Danielle. Her husband Brian and Chris have known each other since high school and became great friends over the last twelve or so years. I always enjoyed his wife's company when we hung out. Their son battled leukemia as a small child and made it through so she had an idea of what I was about to go through. Her email was light, funny, and to the point. She was volunteering to take me to all my chemotherapy treatments and listed her qualifications as:

Being able to sit next to me quietly.

Being able to talk all day if I needed it.

Help me with anything medical without getting grossed out.

> *She said she had more than enough vacation days available and her boss was very understanding.*
>
> *Also she was able to drive while someone was puking into a bag next to her.*

I laughed so hard at her last comment about the driving and puking, yet not really understanding it.

CHAPTER ELEVEN

PAY ATTENTION DAMN-IT!

The morning of my port surgery was very similar to my first surgery. I had gone for a consultation the day before this outpatient surgery and the physician's assistant who was supposed to explain the surgery to me instead questioned me on my family history, cancer and how I found out I had cancer. She said she was 'interested' in this type of thing. Being a talker, I blabbed on about everything that happened, relishing the attention. The Other had always warned other people about attention, speaking to what he knew, playing music.

"Attention," he would say. *"is very addictive. You must be careful or you can get carried away by it and miss the whole point in what you are there to do. Attention from other people can wreck a relationship. It can cost you your job. It can ruin your life if you are not careful with it."* Always reiterating at the end, *"I cannot stress this enough; attention is highly addictive."*

I fell right into it. This P.A. was asking about me and my life and family and instead of me questioning what was going to be happening; I got off course and answered her questions, instead of her mine. I kept no focus. I had been alone in our home for the past couple of weeks about eleven hours a day while Chris worked and made the long drive both ways. I was desperate for adult interaction—something I was used to on a daily basis.

At the end of our conversation, she quickly ran through what my port would be doing, and how they 'installed' it. It seemed fairly simple and handy. She told me:

"Instead of having to have blood draws through your arm, they will all go through the port now, if you ever had an IV, it could be run through the port."

I was happy. I knew my dad's arms were bruised and battered.

His veins were starting to collapse because of all the blood draws. It wasn't until later when I spoke to Danielle (the friend who sent the email about her qualifications for taking me to chemotherapy) that I actually did learn how a port was supposed to work for the chemo. A question I realized later that I didn't ask and have wondered to this day why the 'consultation' with this P.A. didn't volunteer the information.

Here I was, having talked to both an oncology nurse and a P.A. neither of whom made an effort to explain anything except their own personal feelings. Once again, without me knowing it, I was unprepared for what was to follow.

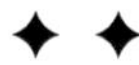

I had to learn to let others take the lead, not pay attention so much to details, I had to let myself be sick. Chris's mom was taking me on all these little trips back and forth to the hospital. I loved the fact that she was able to do all this stuff for me, and she was good on the phone. She was able to call and talk to people and cut through the crap that I would get frustrated with. Although, I couldn't help but wish my dad wasn't sick so he and my mom could take me. My dad understood medical jargon and was comfortable in hospitals. I wanted my mom there to talk to and tell me it would be alright. Even at my age, parents bring a comfort like no one else can, a safety net around you.

Sue parked in valet and got a wheel chair. I am not a small woman, at that time down to 202. I felt very guilty for making Chris's mom push me around, but I couldn't walk. She seemed to know where she was going and wheeled me up to the desk after the elevator ride. We checked in and were told to wait in a small room. There were a few others, a tall thin African-American man who had already changed into the hospital gown, sitting with his clothes in a clear plastic bag. I thought, why are they making him sit here amongst the clothed, and where was his ride? Did someone drop him off? I was worried about how he would get home. There was a frail elderly lady and her loud mouth daughter. Too stupid to get her mother one of the many wheelchairs lined up at all the entrances she was eyeing mine.

After sitting there for 25 minutes past our 'must be there at 7 am arrival,' Sue walked over to the desk.

"It will just be a couple of minutes." I could hear the girl say in a dismissive tone.

An aide arrived in the room and took away the other people which was a welcome relief as the daughter would not get off her phone and was speaking loudly about what amounted to a conversation that could easily have taken place after all the patients were in surgery and she could step outside. I am all for instant communication, and had she been instructing her children in her absence, or giving an update on her mother's condition, I would have been more tolerant, but seriously, a conversation about reality TV or what you ate last night, that's who those large signs about cell phone use in doctor's offices and Hospitals are directed to. "PLEASE TURN OFF CELL PHONES."

Finally, at 7:35 am an aide stepped into the room and called my name. I don't know who she was directing the call out to, as everyone else was gone. It could not have given me less encouragement to know that the hospital worker couldn't tell the difference between the upright woman in the chair reading (Chris's mom) and the slumped over woman in the wheelchair with her feet propped on a chair, no makeup, hair pulled back, in pajama bottoms and tennis shoes (me).

She took me into what looked like a plain department store changing room from the 1970's. Showed me how to lift the lids on the wooden seats and pointed out the small, medium, and large hospital gowns, handed me the plastic bag and explained the process for disrobing. I grabbed two gowns and the socks and headed into the first curtained room. Changing and carefully folding my clothes, I headed back to the outer room and sat back in the wheel chair. The aide pushed me down a hall. Sue came with me holding the plastic bag.

The fact that the stupid bag they gave you irritated me again. While in the hospital on several different appointments I saw many family member walking around with them. Clothes all jammed in. I thought to myself if I have to do this again I'm going to bring some bright neon underwear and bras and place them on the outside of my clothes, not discreetly rolled up within my pj bottoms. Or maybe some wild leopard print. Large, clear bags offer people very little in the way of modesty.

We went to a nicer waiting room, and of course we waited again. At 8 am, a plain clothed hospital worker came out and asked if I was Kimberly. Since I was the only one in the waiting room with a hospital gown on, it was the logical conclusion once again not bolstering my confidence in anyway. She wheeled me into a small office and took down all the necessary info so they could get paid. She asked if anyone explained the procedure, more as a statement then a question, and never waited for an answer before calling for another aide to come and get me. The aide wheeled me off *sans* Sue into a very small operating room. A male nurse came in and took some vitals. He got me a warm blanket saying the doctors liked to keep the rooms colder. A second female nurse came in to start the IV. She had a hard time and had to pull up a chair and sit down and relax herself before it worked. I think more embarrassed by her lack of skills, she left the room immediately. I sat there for a while by myself looking around. I was displeased to see the amount of dust that had collected on the plastic covered wires and computer screens. In fact, the screens on the equipment looked like DOS from the 1980's. I was surprised that no one had weighed me or asked me my weight. When IV nurse was searching for a vein, she explained exactly what was going to happen and asked a lot of questions about my surgery and my personal life. She said the appropriate, "*oh I'm sorry*" at the diagnosis question but followed with a story of how easy chemo would be, and I could still probably make my wedding on August 28th in Vegas. Upon her return to the room, she asked me to climb onto a table and lay flat on my back. She and the male nurse did their best to prop me up in a comfortable way. I needed to lay on my back for the surgery but that wasn't happening because of the last surgery. So a series of wedges and pillows placed under and around me helped with my comfort.

She started the medicine in the IV and said I would get very relaxed and sleepy but would probably not be totally asleep–although if I felt like it to go ahead and sleep. I felt the medicine start to work; I relaxed. *I could sleep,* I thought and tried to drift off.

The doctor arrived and through his mask introduced himself. He spoke kindly and asked if I felt relaxed. I did and told him so. He told me he would have me out in a jiffy and said:

"Now, I'm going to give you a shot." He placed his finger below my collar bone on the right side. He was honest and said *"This is gonna sting like the dickens but it will numb the area fast."*

He put the needle in, and I said, *"You're right. It hurts but not as bad as my other surgery."*

I started to drift off. I didn't feel the incision being made, and I thought of the time I woke up while my wisdom tooth was being pulled; you're sleepy, but nothing hurts, so you don't care. Then, I felt it... something being pushed into my body. I spoke up,

"*I can feel that.*"

"*You can?*" The doctor sounded bewildered.

The insertion halted as the doctor spoke to the nurse who put the IV in. "*Push fifty more cc's.*"

"*Yes doctor.*"

There was silence for a few moments...

The pushing into my body started again. A searing pain in the right clavicle area as if a hot knife was being pushed into my body.

"*I can still feel that*"

"*Push twenty more cc's.*"

"*Pushing twenty more.*"

Silence again, and then the pain started. Now I was irritated and wide awake.

"*Seriously people! I CAN FEEL THAT!!*"

"*Ok Kim,*" the doctor said in hushed tones. *"We're almost done."*

The pain intensified. I felt the slicing through the underside of my skin. It burned and hurt. I could feel myself getting more and more upset. What the hell is wrong with these people in this hospital?! No one listening to or believing me!

"*THAT HURTS!!*" In the loudest tone I could get out.

"*Ok Kim we are almost done.*" The doctor's tone was the same, hushed and calm.

I felt the male nurse grab my hand. "*Squeeze my hand if you need to.*" He tried to distract me...

"So tell me about the wedding on a pirate ship in Vegas you are planning..."

The doctor mumbled something to the IV nurse and I heard movement. The male nurse continued in a calming tone.

"I went to my cousin's wedding out in Vegas. What a great place. I couldn't figure out what to do first. It's so busy. Now the doc's going to stitch you up real quick."

The doctor now used the same happy tone as his male nurse.

"It's only gonna take a few stitches. How you holding up Kim?"

The burning, cutting, and pushing had stopped although the area was now throbbing.

"The area is throbbing," I managed to say in a not so irritated tone.

"I'm all done. Sorry about that. Good luck to you," he said a few medical things to the two people in the room and left.

'Sorry about that?' Well at least this time I received a half-hearted apology. However, I was angry about my treatment.

Two more people entered the room. They came with a different gurney and the four of them slowly helped me slide from one table to another. The two nurses that had been with me said good luck and with that the new people rolled me out the door and to post-op.

This area was a little different than the post-op before. There was more room in the curtained area, or maybe there were less machines and people. There was a chair and Sue came in and sat down.

The nurse in post-op took my vitals and looked at a computer screen. She propped me up a little and brought me juice and graham crackers. The diet of cancer people and post-surgery victims in this hospital. I managed over the next hour to get down four crackers and two containers of juice. I finally sat up and got myself dressed with some assistance.

The aide helped me to the wheel chair and rolled me to the valet entrance with Sue. We waited for our car for what seemed like an eternity.

It was lunch time and people were coming and going. I noticed many doctors, nurses and other hospital workers using valet. I was waiting watching the beautiful, sunshiny Michigan day. The houses backing up to the hospital were lined with beautiful flowers and trees.

A landscaping company tended to the grass on hospital property. The buffer zone, I'm sure meant to obstruct the view of the enormous buildings, was only about fifty feet wide, and then there was the main hospital road; four lanes wide and a steady stream of traffic.

I watched the valet guys get stuck in lunch-hour traffic. I sat there sick to my stomach, upper chest throbbing, still not in even fifty percent from my last surgery, waiting and waiting more than fifteen minutes later I saw Sue's truck and the end of the line of cars, it would be four more minutes till it got to me.

The hundreds of cars every Friday and Saturday night didn't have to wait this long, I thought of my old friend and his valet company. He needs this account I thought. Five dollars a car, it's busy nonstop, and you only have two people working. Idiots!

I was able to call Chris on the ride home. It was twelve-thirty. I had been up since 6a.m. I was exhausted, but the sound of Chris's voice made me feel better.

As we headed down the back roads because the main expressway, and shortest route, was under construction, I started to notice how much brighter everything seemed to look, even the dinginess of the closed buildings, in one industrial park after another, seemed to glow as the weeds of the unkempt driveways and parking-lots sparkled in green and vibrant wild flowers. The State of Michigan and its residents were suffering badly, and all this had taken its toll on our many commercial buildings, and yet under the layer of grime I could somehow see beauty where I once saw blight.

"You don't need to kick the crap out of someone. You don't need to scratch your nails on a chalkboard. You want to torture someone, yeah, put them in charge of their own survival. Then treat them with chemotherapy."

- Richard S., Fourth round chemotherapy patient.

CHAPTER TWELVE

COMMUNICATION IS A PROBLEM

The date for the first round of chemotherapy was fast approaching. In the fifteen days between the installation of the port and the first chemo, I had two more blood draws and finally a visit with the doctor. When I walked into his office on the third of August, it had been twenty days since I had seen him and heard his diagnosis in the late afternoon on the day of my surgery.

I sat for over an hour in the waiting room and another twenty five minutes in the exam room. This time, I sat solo, not wanting a reoccurrence of the crying and passing out from the last office visit. The doctor walked through the door upbeat and sincere, sat next to me in a chair, and read the exact diagnosis from the lab. He was correct in his Stage III Ovarian Cancer. It was marked 3B and noted as 'bulky'. The doctor explained what A,B,C meant in the one through four staging of cancers. In simple terms, one is the least and four is the most, and A is the least with C being the most. Effectively, there are actually twelve stages of cancers, with each of the four main stages being broken down farther into three parts. Is there a vast difference between these three extra parts the stages are broken down into? Doctors will tell you yes. It makes a difference in what treatment is ordered. However, I have talked to many with Stage III Ovarian Cancer diagnosed around the same time as me, and we were all given the same chemotherapy drugs in intervals of three or four weeks, no matter if we were A, B or C attached to the number three.

My doctor said that I would need six rounds of chemotherapy, and then I would meet with him again to see if I might need two more. He told me that my treatment would be monitored by his oncology nursing staff, and that I would not need to talk to him again until the end of treatment- adding, that if I got a call to see him, it would only be for bad news. Then, he asked if I had questions. This time I actually did. Having randomly gone to 'chemotherapy' sites and 'cancer' sites by googling these two words, the same types of things kept coming up. In fact, many of them with the exact same verbiage; I thought to myself, this can't be too bad. The play down of the treatment set me at ease. However, I wanted to double check.

I had to ask first, *"What are my chances of getting through this and getting rid of it completely?"* I remember asking about my chances in the hospital, but I wanted confirmation of what he had already said.

"About 80/20," he said seriously. *"This treatment works in about 80%, and they come out on the other side golden."*

I took that statement to mean 'cured,' and he added no extra information to that statement. No alternatives, no additional treatments, just flat out–it either works or it doesn't. That is what I took to heart. I had the feeling that 80% was a high number, and since I made it through the surgery, I felt I was a good candidate for making it through this.

"What kind of side-effects can I expect?" Was the next thing out of my mouth.

"Well, have you gone on-line and looked them up?" The doc asked in response.

"Yes." I had googled chemotherapy. I did not have the exact name of the medicine that would be used on me. I didn't say that however, and the doctor didn't clarify.

"Well." And here it was again *"Everybody's different. I would expect to experience everything, and if you don't, good for you."*

Looking back with more information, and more experience, I can't tell you how ludicrous that statement was to me. My doctor *told* me *to go look it up on the internet.* When you look at a general list for chemotherapy side-effects, it covers all aspects of all chemotherapy medicines. Each one has its own list of what to expect. My favorite in the list was always—Diarrhea, Constipation. How can you have both? Yet, all lists had both.

"But don't worry" he continued *"We will give you medicines to help with the side-effects. If you need anything ask one of the nurses. They will get it for you. They are very experienced in doing this. They know as much as me*

most times."

"What should I eat, and can I take vitamins or supplements?"

The doctor was quick with a reply. *"Eat whatever you want and can keep down. I want you to eat. I don't want you to lose any weight while you go through this. And no vitamins, no herbs or supplements. Some interfere with your drugs. We don't want that. Wait until you are done with treatment, and then you can take them."*

"Can I go back into the office?" He had already told me before the surgery I could work from home immediately after surgery, and I had begun working from home, but I wanted back into my office ASAP. I was sick of looking at the inside walls of my home.

"I am not going to put any restrictions on you. You do whatever you feel you can do. We will work chemotherapy around your schedule for work. We are open all the time."

On that good bit of news, I wanted him to know what happened with the port surgery, and I relayed the story. Not really knowing what to expect, but I felt he should know that there are others in this hospital network that I felt were not up to the standard he set. It was also going to be in the lead in for what I hoped to be a frank conversation about his nurse that I had already gone head to head with, not just on scheduling but also on my staple removal...

I had stopped on the day before my port surgery to see the nurse that had argued with me on scheduling. She was to remove the staples from surgery. Because they had sliced through my belly button there was also a staple there. Unfortunately for me, I had been blessed with a mole in my belly button. I had had it removed twice in my life, but it kept growing back. As she pulled out the staples, she had also been pulling off scabs to my dismay. I asked her not to remove the scabs but to let them fall off naturally. She scoffed and rolled her eyes. Then I felt her picking at the mole in my belly button. I immediately spoke up.

"I have a mole in my belly button. Please don't touch it. That is not a scab."

"I have to see if there is a stitch under it," she said curtly.

I grabbed her hand and yelled at her, *"DON'T TOUCH IT, I SAID! IT'S A MOLE NOT A SCAB!"*

She looked back at her work and continued silently not touching my belly button again. When she finished, she said, *"When that stitch in your navel becomes infected, you'll have to come back in."*

I must note here, that there wasn't a stitch under my mole, and I never got an infection.

Wanting desperately to let the doctor know about this nurse, I started with the port surgery and what had happened waiting for a reaction of anger that something like that would happen, instead I got…

"I'm sorry you had to go through that, but let me get the girls to get your calendar and get you going." He took my hand in his and stood up. *"It's been an honor and a privilege Kim."* And with that, he left.

His departure was followed by a conversation at the desk where I could hear him directing the girls what to do, and a few minutes later, the aide came in and said I could go to the desk for instructions.

Once at the desk, I was handed a calendar printout of the month of August with the 13th marked with 8 am chemotherapy' and August 10th marked with 'Blood Draw.' I asked if there was a different place to go for the blood draw, since all the previous draws had been done for surgeries in the surgery area of the hospital.

She said, *"Yes, out our door, across the lobby and through the pharmacy."*

"And chemotherapy?" I was so surprised I had to ask about either of these things. I thought that from what I saw on television that the cancer community was this big caring faction of people who guided you through. It actually felt no different than any other doctor's office, like I should just 'know' everything.

"Right down the hall." She pointed in the other direction

Sue, before my first chemotherapy, would go to the hospital and look at the chemotherapy room, so she knew where it was the day of my first treatment.

I directed my next question to the women sitting there that weren't the receptionist, assuming one of them was a nurse of some kind. *"So, how does this port work? I thought it was going to be level with the skin"*

When the P.A. had shown me this little device, it had a round spongy surface connected to a tube. I thought that surface with its quarter-sized white surface would be visible. It was not. It was under the skin and had been stitched closed.

"There is a needle that will be inserted like an IV needle, just a little bigger," said one of the women.

"It is still tender." I related an abbreviated version of the surgery incident.

"I can write you a script for a salve to put on the area if you want," the same woman said.

"I think I'll take that," I said quickly.

As she wrote the script, she explained that the salve should be put on an hour before chemo starts, and don't cover it with a Band-Aid, use Tegaderm.

I nodded that I understood and wrote down the word "Tegaderm."

"Where can I get this 'Tegaderm?" I questioned her.

"The pharmacy should have it."

"Now for nausea and other side effects – do I need any prescriptions for that?"

"We'll give them to you the day of your treatment."

"Ok thanks. I just don't want to throw up." It is what I had feared most in the list of side effects.

"Don't worry. There are a hundred kinds of pills for that."

And with that I left, walked out the door and walked across the lobby to the pharmacy in the hospital figuring they would have this special salve over my normal pharmacy, since the hospital cancer center was right there. They had the salve, not the Tegaderm, but they gave us a place we could go to and get it.

I started to feel my irritation rise with the whole process. I felt as a cancer patient, that I should have been given more information. So far, everything that I knew had come from the internet which I wasn't that comfortable with, and the fact that I had to ask about the port and what to do to prevent more pain made me mad. I was feeling like they should be telling me things, and I shouldn't have to ask because I really had no idea what I should be asking. As we drove to the location that the pharmacy sent us to, I was irritated that the pharmacy didn't have what the patients within the hospital needed.

The building they sent us to was an office that processed the orders for the pharmacy; the pharmacy had told us it was their main warehouse. It was not. No luck. I took two more medical supply stores to finally get this Tegaderm. Five pieces of it was twelve dollars and some change.

Later, I would find out from my friends that were nurses, that what you need is something to keep the glopped on salve from getting all over your clothes and that wouldn't absorb the product. Plastic wrap would work. Again, all the nurses I knew could tell me this, yet no one who was treating me could.

This lack of communication would only get worse.

CHAPTER THIRTEEN
ALL JACKED-IN

I went for my first 'cancer blood draw' not really knowing it at the time, but these numbers would soon start to control me, make me worry and stress out, as they do to many patients.

When I walked into the hospital lab and signed in, the proper paperwork was filled out and I was back in one of two tiny rooms. I immediately mentioned the port remembering that the P.A. had told me that it could be used for blood draws.

"We can't do that," the lady said as she grabbed empty vials out of the drawer next to the chair I was sitting in.

"The lady I talked to the day before the installation of this port said that blood could be drawn from it– I had it done in this hospital," I insisted.

"Honey, you have to be specially trained to do that. Not just anybody can do it. First, you have to be a licensed nurse and then on top of that have special training. We aren't nurses in the lab." She was examining both my arms trying to find a large enough vein.

"Well then, you'll need a butterfly needle to draw blood."

She reached into her drawer and pulled out a different package, throwing the one off the counter back in the drawer. *"Ok, tell me your name and birth date."*

I repeated my name and birthday as she placed labels on all the empty vials. She inserted the needle and filled all the vials seamlessly. I drove thirty-five minutes to get there, and the whole process took less than three minutes, if you don't count the paperwork. Plus, I had to pay for parking and walk in.

I was getting better at walking for longer periods of time, and driving was ok because I was sitting. It was the need to eat and drink every two hours that was throwing me. Because of the surgery and the vast amount of time I spent not eating, followed by the weeks of diarrhea and pain, I couldn't eat like I used to. I would take in four or five ounces of food about every two hours, and if I didn't, I would find myself feeling sick from the hunger. Leaving the house for the hour round trip usually meant I had to bring a bottle of water and those graham crackers they gave out at the hospital to the cancer patients.

Everything I did seemed to take longer and had to be well planned. I was four weeks out of surgery now: the point that I thought I would be able to go back into the office. And yet I was setting up myself for my first chemotherapy treatment. It was now starting to sink in. What I had planned before and right after surgery wasn't going to happen. My bosses had told me I wasn't expected back until after Labor Day, yet after explaining what was going on with me their answer was to work from home on an hourly basis until I was through with the chemo treatments. I was angry. Angry at the cancer for getting in the way of my job. Angry at myself for not 'fixing' this health issue sooner. Angry at the world because this happened to me. It all seemed idiotic. I had been emailing three people who I knew well and who each confided in me the cancer that they had and told no one. They tried to work through all the treatments, telling me, *"I wasn't going to let cancer win."* It didn't seem feasible, and for the first time in my life, I had a boss who was encouraging me to take care of myself. However, I couldn't get over my long held belief that I needed to work full-time, in order to be me.

I was stuck with mounting medical bills and now a major cut in pay. I needed to come to terms with the part-time work from home.

Sue and I walked down the hall from the doctor's office and around the corner and entered another waiting room, signed in, filled out some paperwork and sat down to wait as people were called back. It was Friday August 13th. Just my luck I thought... only I could be unlucky enough to draw my first chemotherapy treatment on Friday the 13th!

They started to call back people who arrived after me. Again Sue had to go to the desk to ask what the problem was.

"Your appointment is at 8:30."

I answered from my chair, *"They told me 8:00."*

"We don't take people in the order they sign in. It's according to what they are having done, so it doesn't matter anyways. We'll call you soon."

They did... at 8:35.

We walked through the side door as instructed and I saw a large room with a nurses' station in the center. Around the outside walls was chair after chair, divided by curtains. There were a few hospital beds at the corners and three private rooms. I was sent to a private room with a large reclining chair. I sat down and got settled. Sue noticed a cart on the way in with juices, coffee and, of course, graham crackers. She went to grab juice and crackers for me and coffee for herself. I missed coffee. After the surgery, I was so sick I didn't drink any, and I had read online that I shouldn't eat or drink anything that 'I love' because it might make me sick and then I wouldn't want to eat or drink my favorites at the end of treatment. With that in mind I choose not to drink coffee for a while.

One of the three nurses working about twenty-five chairs and beds came into my room and removed the Tegaderm from my clavicle; she took out a sponge from a plastic seal which had a self-feeding alcohol stick on it. She used the sponge to remove the thick white paste and disinfect the area around the port. She then took another fairly large needle out of plastic which was connected to a piece of clear plastic about two inches long. I turned my head in the other direction as I knew what was coming next

"Ok," my nurse started to talk. *"Take a really deep breath. I'm going to count to three and then exhale."*

On the exhale, she inserted the needle through the skin and into the port. There was a sharp prick, but I believed the numbing cream was working and it was pretty tolerable. This insertion into my port was followed by drawing blood out of the port. Good blood return, I would come to understand in later months is essential to that port working correctly. Once she established that she had blood flow, she hooked the insert to a saline IV line. I was officially 'all jacked-in.' A term I decided to use because the chemotherapy port reminded me of the movie *The Matrix*. I thought that this little line of chemicals would transport me back to my healthy self. Back to my life. Back to being Kim, and not Kim with cancer. Frankly, Kim with cancer was a pain in my ass! She had taken away fun Kim.

Because it was my first visit into that cancer center, there was paperwork as usual- looking for all the stats so the hospital can be paid.

Nobody asked how I was feeling. Nobody questioned anything actually.

At this particular cancer center, once you are hooked to an IV, your medicine is ordered from the hospital pharmacy. Since I had spoken with the doctor so recently, everything was in the computer, and about an hour later, the medicine showed up.

I used that hour to force my story on the nurse that was taking care of me. I don't know if she wanted to hear it, but I was going to make sure that the list of side effects I had looked up on line were covered like I had asked. So as IV bags started to be hung and connected to my working port, I was asked my name and birth date. In return, I asked the name of the drug, what it was for, how long it would take to be administered, and then I used my laptop to Google the drug and find out the side effects.

My treatment went like this:

Decadron– Steroid- for side-effects - 15 minutes
Aloxi—a long release (5day) anti-nausea med - 30 minutes
Benadryl—for side effects – pushed through a needle into the IV - 1minute
Zofran – anti-nausea med – 30 minutes
Taxol -chemotherapy—3 hours
Flush line—15 minutes
Carboplatin—chemotherapy–1.5 hours
Flush line—15 minutes

As these medicines were being pushed into my body for the first time they really didn't bother me, except for the Benadryl- which completely surprised me. I had taken Benadryl hundreds of times, mostly for severe allergy/hay fever outbreaks at night. It would dry up my sinuses and knock me out. I expected the same thing. Only that isn't what happened.

I started to get that medicine head feeling. I set aside my computer thinking I would fall asleep. Instead my legs began to twitch in different random ways. I felt tired enough but couldn't fall asleep. Instead I sat back in the recliner feeling waves of swimming incoherentness, with legs moving about, and an occasional swell of being sick to my stomach. It lasted about an hour and slowly tapered off. I asked the nurse about it, and she said that next time she would ask the pharmacy to "piggyback" the med in saline solution so that it could be administered slowly. After that first round, Benadryl was given to me in that form and took about fifteen minutes to pump into my body. The side-effects were less severe but they were noticeable.

The three nurses that worked in this center moved all day long. I never saw one of them sit down, drink a glass of water, or chat with each other unless it was directly related to a patient in the center. They worked so well as a team, and each of them answered any and all questions I had, to what I feel was the best of their abilities. I thought they were incredibly patient, understanding, and informative (when asked). They didn't complain. I had known all nurses worked hard. I had never watched an entire shift work together like this, with every chair and bed being full all day long.

As I sat there all day doing my drug research, the doctor's office assistant stopped by to see me. She gave me a 'chemo calendar.' On it was the date of my current chemo and arrival time, my next chemo and arrival time and two dates for blood draws. My chemo month would look like this:

- Week One: Friday- Chemotherapy
- Week Three: Thursday—Blood Draw at Lab
- Week Four: Tuesday—Blood Draw at Lab
- Week Four: Friday-Chemotherapy

Meaning in four weeks' time, I would be at the hospital four times, twice all day, and twice to have blood drawn.

This center was twenty minutes from my home (thirty-five in summer construction traffic) and it cost three dollars to park each time.

A short while after the office assistant stopped by, the oncology nurse came with a prescription for Zofran pills. I was instructed to start taking them exactly eight hours apart until Monday morning. Right after she left the nurse in the cancer center said that if I still felt sick on Monday I could take them a day or two longer and then a statement that would haunt me:

"Don't ever let yourself get ***behind*** *the nausea or pain."*

I asked what she meant.

"When you are taking these, take them on time. Not like people do with antibiotics, you know. The label says three times a day, so they take them at breakfast, lunch, and dinner. Don't do that. Work your schedule out, so you take them exactly eight hours apart. When Monday comes and you get to that eight hour mark and start to feel a little sick to your stomach, take another pill. Don't just stop. When you can get to eight or nine hours and you aren't feeling sick to your stomach, then you stop."

She paused to make sure I understood, and I had to ask what would happen if I stopped too soon.

"If you stop too soon and get sick, then it is hard to go back."

Now, in my head, I totally understood that statement. My body was a different story.

"You won't have to worry too much because your IV anti-nausea medicine will last five days."

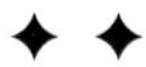

At the end of all these drugs flowing into my body and the nurses instructions, we headed home. Sue filled my scripts at the local pharmacy and was on her way home. I set myself up on the couch to read more about the drugs. They all said the same exact thing:

- *Tiredness*
- *Nausea*
- *Constipation*
- *Diarrhea*

Then there was what I thought would be the scary stuff:

- *Hair loss*

- *Loosening of the nail beds*
- *Mouth sores*
- *Numbness of extremities*

There were warnings on the websites about things to call your doctor or go to the emergency room for. I felt prepared, and with the nurses assuring me about the anti-nausea meds, I thought I could handle anything.

I can honestly say after the events following my surgery, I felt like it couldn't get any worse than what I had been through. And although just days in my past, I was already beginning to forget what that type of hurt and humiliation felt like. I came home feeling tired but not over-whelmed and thought I was treated pretty well.

What I didn't see at this cancer center was all the love and camaraderie that I thought went with this illness. You see it on TV: people joining together, helping, volunteering. I only saw paid employees and the occasional family member. In fact, many of the people were dropped off or walked in of their own accord. Only a few people had someone with them all day long like I did. I thought, *Well it would be like me to end up in a center where there was no support or help.* I made a note to myself to ask next month, during my treatment, where I could find support for myself. I wasn't sure what that was going to encompass, and I was hoping it would mean I could get a little financial help, but at this point I needed to get the ball rolling in one direction or another.

"We are all the same inside these four walls of the infusion center. There is no race, religion or politics to separate us. Just the difference between the sick and the well."

~Madilynne Crosse,
Seventeen rounds of chemotherapy.
Three year cervical cancer survivor.

CHAPTER FOURTEEN

THE TRUTH: LIKE NO ONE ELSE WILL EVER EXPLAIN IT TO YOU

If you read no other chapter in this book except this one, I personally would be a happy camper. In all my rantings of the many things I didn't do for my own health, it really all comes down to this...

You can read these next pages and know that if I could reverse anything it would be that I was more patient in my life and that I went to the same doctor on a regular basis. That after my grandmother's and great aunt's deaths, I would have done much more research on the types of cancer they had when it came to genetic lines. I should also mentions, when my grandmother and aunt passed, the internet as we know it didn't exist, so research really required good old-fashioned leg work.

I believe I was destined to get Ovarian Cancer no matter what I would have done, but I think I could have caught it much, much earlier and prevented the long duration of what I am about to explain. In other words, the following could not have been avoided, but perhaps I would have had less treatments, and longer remissions in between.

The hard fact of all this is that the next chapter is not going to be easy to read. It comes with all types of warnings from me. I don't recommend reading this chapter on your lunch hour if you have a week stomach or in a crowded place if you embarrass easily. I looked everywhere for this type of information and only came up with these 'words':

- *Constipation*
- *Diarrhea*
- *Joint Pain*
- *Nausea*

- *Altered Taste*
- *Neuropathy*

Nowhere did anyone actually explain these words... as they relate to chemotherapy.

Ah, but you say, Kim we know what constipation means... you know, when you can't poop. Cancer constipation is nothing like that. Everyone has bouts of constipation in their life or even live with it-only pooping as few as a couple of times a week. Still not the same as you will soon read.

I have chosen to not use medical terminology in this section. Bowel Movement or BM will be replaced by words like poop and shit. Why? Because it is the way we actually think and talk. When you 'medical up' statements I don't believe them to have the same effect on the human brain. When you call your mom looking for sympathy you don't say—"the kids were nauseous all night long" you say- "the kids puked all over their beds and me, there is a trashcan full of shitty diapers—I'm exhausted".

It will all be here for you... in easy to understand language.

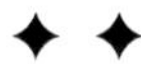

Because of the steroids administered by IV, I didn't sleep for the first two nights. Still recovering from surgery, I wasn't able to move around much, but mentally I was wide awake. The feeling of being sick-to-my-stomach started to creep in on the second day. It started almost as an overly-hungry feeling. If you have ever gone over a day without eating, you might have experienced this feeling. You get sick-to-your-stomach usually combined with a massive headache and think to yourself, *if I don't eat soon I'm going to puke.* Another relative symptom to draw off is the feeling you might get with a migraine where you are sick to your stomach with a headache. Many women also get this feeling into their forties with their menstrual cycles—a sickness in the lower abdomen accompanied by headache.

I was on top of things but paranoid about vomiting. I set my phone to go off at exactly eight hours to take my anti-nausea pill. With that said, on the first day out of chemo, I was three pills into the routine when I noticed at about the six-hour mark I was starting to feel really sick. I managed to hold off till seven hours, and without authorization, I took my medicine. I reset my phone for eight hours again, and again, this time at the six hour mark, feeling even sicker, and I took my pill early.

I managed to eat something small about every two hours. I was told 'to eat whatever I could keep down' by the doctor and took advantage of that, eating things that I had not eaten in years. Always kind of keeping my intake to 2-4ounces of anything I ate. I drank a ton of water, and a limited amount of Hawaiian Punch. I don't know why I wanted that particular drink since I hadn't had it since I was a child at my grandmother's house, but it 'sounded' good.

And, I did have strange cravings and went with each of them. I was actually happy with my water intake, managing to get in about two quarts a day which was very unusual for me. I had never been a big water drinker.

As Saturday turned to Sunday, the uncontrollable sickness deep within my stomach, lower abdomen and now inching up into my chest managed to intensified with each pill. Topped off by the fact that the duration the pill would last was shortening. By Sunday night, the pill was only keeping off the nausea by about four hours, and I was waiting seven hours to take it. I hadn't pooped since Thursday morning, and it was now about 6pm on Sunday.

Hoping to get my mind off things with some adult-style cartoons on Sunday night TV, I asked Chris to help me get set up in our bed. I still couldn't sleep lying down; however, Chris's mom had brought over foam wedges to help prop me up.

Chris got me set up with my legs also propped with a big foam wedge under my knees, and slowly over the next two hours, I became increasingly more uncomfortable. My legs felt like they had a combination of growing pains and the after-effects of too much exercise/muscle strain. My hips were in a tremendous amount of arthritic-type pain; my body became increasing restless and started moving about. The pain increased tenfold over the next four hours and was unrelenting.

I lay in our bed squirming, moving desperately trying to get relief. It became like a thousand knives poking me over and over again. Chris sat in a folding chair next to the bed trying anything he could think of to move or adjust things to help me. After four hours, I lost it and began to cry, not only was the pain there, but the nausea was coming back. The fierceness of it was unrelenting. I asked for help to get into the bathroom, and as I sat down on the toilet I could feel the churning inside of me, the lightheadedness that comes with vomiting. I stood up to turn around and lift the seat of the toilet and started to vomit, and as I did I felt pee pouring down my leg, with each guttural heave more pee spilled from me. I reached for the garbage can and put it under me to catch what I could, while reaching around for towels from behind me to drop on the floor and absorb the urine that was soaking the floor tiles.

Our bathroom is only 6 x 8, with a straight layout of door, sink, toilet and then the tub running perpendicular in the six foot direction.

I panicked as I watched the neon green bile come up. I flushed as often as the toilet would let me. My throat burned; my mouth burned; my legs were in pain still and now feeling raw from the pee that was soaking into both of them. I stopped vomiting for a moment and turned to sit down again on the toilet, dumping the wastepaper basket, its urine soaked paper contents and what pee it caught into the tub next to me.

I yelled for Chris who had been outside the closed door, but as the door opened I started to heave again. The metal wastepaper basket smelled and made me gag more. I yelled:

"Get me another garbage can!" In my head, I thought the plastic garbage can in my office, however the closest garbage can was in our room and it was wicker! Chris handed me the wicker garbage can and I threw it back at him and barked,

"Get me a bucket" which he immediately retrieved. Had it been me, I would have probably left at that moment.

Here was this great guy, holding my hand through my misery and I was out of control, panicking and yelling things.

He handed me the bucket and said,

"Don't worry about the mess. I will clean it up when you are done."

I'm sure it must have been a mess looking in. Wet garbage in the tub, all the towels crumpled and wet on the floor, and the smell...Pee and vomit.

I started again uncontrollably vomiting into the bucket. It hurt to sit on the toilet upright. The pains in my side were getting worse. I couldn't seem to stop heaving, over and over until there was nothing left in my stomach, and I couldn't figure out where all this pee was coming from.

I managed to stop myself from heaving long enough to stand up and wash my mouth out with an antiseptic rinse and then water over and over. I left my pee soaked pajama bottoms on the floor and threw my pajama tops on the floor also. I walked back into the bedroom and grabbed my terrycloth robe, wiped off and put new pajamas on, all while Chris cleaned up my mess.

I lay back down on the bed and immediately had to get back up. I went to the bathroom sat down again on the toilet and started vomiting into the bucket. It felt like the lining of my stomach was coming up. I was shaking and in pain. This went on all through the night and into the next day. Eventually, there was nothing left in my stomach or bladder and it was dry heaves and if you can comprehend this, it was dry peeing- you could feel the muscles release and push but nothing would come out. Anything I sipped came back up. There was no eating at all.

Now you might think, like when you have the stomach flu, food poisoning, or a heavy night of drinking, that once you throw up you will get a reprieve for about forty minutes and then start again. However, that is not the way it works with chemotherapy. Once this type of vomiting starts, there is no stop point; it continues on and on. What you have to do is mentally try to stop or, at the very least, do what I did and trust the fact that that even though you were having the heaving sensations, that you could do other things.

At one of my stopping points in the evening, I lay on the bed Chris holding my hand, and I said,

"I can't do this."

He was so patient and kind.

"Yes you can. I know you can. I need you here with me."

"I can't, I can't do this five more times."

"You've come this far. The doctor saved your life in surgery. You can."

"No, I can't."

"Please, I will help you. You can do this."

"I don't know how anyone does this. Why didn't anyone tell me?" I was crying by now and so was Chris.

"I don't know but I know if anyone can, you can," he said through his tears.

"I can't. I can't. I don't get it. I have the highest tolerance for pain of anyone I know. I worked through a wisdom tooth being pulled; remember when I almost sliced through my finger? I just taped it up and never went to the doctor? Why the hell am I in so much pain and so sick? I thought the medicine would help! I can't even imagine NOT having the medicine!"

All those poor people fighting for life who came before the side-effect medicines were available, how the hell did they do it? I really had always sucked it up when it came to being sick. I Went to work, fulfilled my obligations, got it done, and pushed the pain and uncomfortable feelings aside. This was completely different. Unlike nothing I had ever experienced. It made you want to shut your eyes and never wake up again. It was not of this world. The pain was more severe than arthritis or slicing yourself open. The vomiting and sickness in the stomach area more horrific than any flu or hangover. It was all debilitating.

"We'll call the doctor tomorrow, unless you want to go to the hospital tonight."

I asked him at that point if he remembered the movie about the cancer patient that Julie Roberts took care of.

"Dying Young."

"He went through stuff like this, remember? I actually think this is normal. What I don't get is why didn't they warn me."

"I don't know."

"They acted like all this pills would handle this if I followed the instructions!"

And the conversation repeated itself… all night long… the same thoughts, the same questions… all with no answers. I felt I was lost in some other reality, getting sick over and over with no end in sight. I knew I couldn't ever go through this again, and I had already made up my mind.

✦ ✦

When I knew the doctor's office was open, I called and said I needed to talk to the nurse- oncologist. They put me on with the irritating nurse that I had been dealing with. I told her what had been going on all night.

"I guess you could take a Motrin for the pain, but it will go away. Are you eating?"

"I was until yesterday when I started vomiting."

"You need to eat. You'll feel better."

"I can't eat I need to stop vomiting."

"Are you taking your pill RIGHT ON TIME?"

She emphasized it like I didn't understand instructions.

"Yes, but I am getting sick at the four hour mark."

"That's not possible," she said with disdain.

I hung up.

An hour later I called back and told the lady who answers the phone that I want to talk to someone and not–I gave her the name—I said I was done with her and wanted someone else. She gave me someone else to talk to. I explained the whole ordeal in the way this other nurse had treated me.

"I'm done. Fix this NOW!"

"Ok, I'm going to try. You are behind the nausea and pain now, but we'll try to get in front of it."

She asked me if I had any painkillers left from the surgery. I told her I had the Motrin 600. She said to take that and she was going to call me in another anti-nausea pill and another pain killer. Take it for a day or two until you aren't getting sick between pills and stagger the anti-nausea meds. I thanked her and gave her the name of my pharmacy. It was now 10 am, and she said to give her an hour to get the script called in. I hung up and called Chris's mom.

"I need you to go to the pharmacy and get these new pills."

"Ok, I will."

At 1 pm, I called her again wondering where she was. She had errands to run and lived an hour from us.

"I can't wait any longer."

I hung up and called Chris at work. I was angry again, I am not sure if it was the menopause or the fact that I was now laying on the bathroom floor too weak to walk back and forth from the couch or the bed. I wished I had asked Chris to stay home with me. All this confirmed that if I got through this, I wasn't going to do it again.

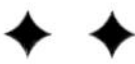

Chris's mom finally showed up with the prescription. Her living so far from us, and having other people to take care of beside me, was compounded by the fact that the chain pharmacy I had the nurse call into hadn't even begun to fill the script by the time she got there. Now even though I had started the processes of trying to get myself right I had wasted another four hours waiting on nurses and pharmacies. When the pills finally arrived I took them right away. Vowing that as soon as I could move I would handle all this crap myself and not depend on anyone else.

I had managed to get myself back to the couch when I knew Sue was on her way. I didn't want her to see me lying on the bathroom floor. After she arrived I sat on the couch I noticed the boredom in Chris's mom. It was hard for her to sit still. She needed something to do.

As a side note, to anyone who wants to assist someone who is having any type of health crisis, let me share something that I was taught early on in my working career. As my work lead me into the management end of hospitality, I learned from a wonderful manager named Dan that to be an effective manager you have to carry out what the owner or corporation wants. He told me that my opinions are always welcome, but to be great at what you do, that your opinions have to follow what the owners are looking to achieve. I remember those words and used them in meetings and interviews. It was my job as a manager to carry out what the owner needs. It really is good advice and carries down even to the hourly employee position. With that said, as someone who is caring for a cancer patient or any patient for that matter, you should think the same way. If your thing is cleaning and you volunteer to clean, then ask, *"Is there a certain way you want his done?"* If you are good at cooking don't just show up with lasagna, ask *"is there something I can make you?"*

A woman from work prepared a week's worth of food for Chris following my surgery and again for a few weeks after my first chemo. She volunteered and asked what I would like. She offered several suggestions of her own and added to my list. But she asked, and that is the important part. I must mention—Chris ate great those weeks. She sent chicken piccata, roasted pork tenderloins, seasoned roasted potatoes, homemade mac and cheese, and some bakery rolls that she remembered I had mentioned that I like. She brought it all over in Glad-Ware containers so it could be frozen or used immediately (and no containers to worry about returning). I remember wishing that I could at least sample some of it. Now, we also had other well-meaning people drop off food, mostly lasagna, none of which we could eat, because they were made with ingredients that either Chris or I didn't like. One phone call could have cleared that up. Just because your family loves it, doesn't mean someone else's family will. Not all families eat onions or mushrooms, some have food allergies or picky eaters. Some eat meat, others don't.

I believe it is so important that as a society we have to help each other, but our help should be based on a genuine need and done out of the goodness in our hearts. You cannot say to yourself:

- *"I'm doing this or that, and they should appreciate it."*
- *"They'll eat what I make."*
- *"They'll owe me after this."*

If you cannot do things from your heart, because you want to, with no thought about 'how much you are owed' then step away. Because what you are actually doing is taking up a lot of space for your own benefit, to make yourself feel less guilty, and the person who is in need of assistance is the one that pays the price; you are there to help them, not to do it your way.

Now of course, it goes without saying that if you ask someone how they want something done and their response is "I don't care" or "it doesn't matter" then this is a person who doesn't want to make a decision or things don't bother them, then take the lead and do what needs to be done, not what you think, what they need. This takes a little thought and common sense. Just because you prefer to clean the bathroom and you are good at it doesn't mean the four days of dirty dishes left by the ailing person's family shouldn't be attended to. You have to help where it is needed the most.

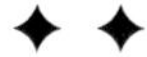

The second pill 'Compazine' kicked in about an hour after Sue brought it over and I took it. The heaving ended and I came to a point I started to call 'chemo coma.' I guess you could say it was medicine head on steroids. Not as bad as the Benadryl push, because I didn't have the twitching, but that loopy, incoherent feeling took over me. I felt like I needed to sleep, which was a relief. I set my alarm for the next pills, carefully spacing out at four hour intervals every other pill. After setting all that up on the calendar on my phone, I went to sleep. And from that Monday until Friday, I felt like I slept more than I was awake. Chris would keep me up to eat and drink. I didn't feel like I could talk in what I would consider normal sentences. I couldn't remember anything, and all my limbs felt heavy, but I wasn't vomiting anymore.

As the days passed, I tried to determine a good day to stop taking the pills. On Friday, eight days from me receiving chemo, I lagged the pills out to five hours apart. I seemed to handle it well; on Saturday I stopped the Compazine in the evening and woke up Sunday to find my chemo coma was gone. I continued the Zofran on Sunday and Monday, stretching the time in between pills out farther and farther. By Tuesday, I had taken one at 5am, and didn't feel sick again until about 5pm. I took my last Zofran on that treatment on Tuesday night. I woke up Wednesday morning and didn't feel sick to my stomach- thirteen days from the administration of my chemotherapy, which brought on a new side-effect; I hadn't pooped since the morning before my chemotherapy fourteen days earlier. In the week on the Compazine, I didn't even know I hadn't gone, being so out of it. I decided I hated that feeling that the Compazine inflicted on me. It was like someone drugged me, so I wouldn't know what was going on. It seemed stupid. I like to be in control. However, it was a small price to pay to not vomit.

The pooping started on Thursday morning (fourteen days after chemotherapy). It was like the surgery all over again. It hurt. My bowels started to move and small little hard pieces would only come out. Most of them I had to dig out with my finger as my rectum wouldn't push them all the way out. For two days, all day long, I would walk back and forth to the bathroom when the pain hit, and bear down, reach around with a piece of toilet paper and reach into my ass and pull out a small chunk of poop. It was such a relief with each piece, and the pain would subside for a short time. On Saturday morning, I had my first really good shit in sixteen days. To say it was *huge* is an understatement. I took a stick, actually it was a small piece of quarter round I found in the basement, to break the poop apart. For a couple of reasons, first, I didn't want to clog the toilet and second, I wanted to see what I was dealing with. It was rock-hard, and took some effort to break up, but there was no blood or mucus, and I thought that was a good thing. I am not sure why I thought to look for those things, but for some reason, when I saw the size of this thing, I thought hemorrhoids... *Because what I really needed was more issues at this point *insert sarcastic tone**... I wasn't feeling very confident in my health, in fact I was the most negative I have ever been in my life.

I pooped about the same amount/size twice more that day. Each time was wonderful. I felt such relief and release in my body. It was amazing that going poop, something I had done every morning for my entire life, would please me so much. I googled the intestines, mostly because I wanted to know how long they were. I had heard all kinds of things about how many feet, but I wanted to know. The answer amazed me and I figured in those two plus weeks I had backed into and filled every inch of the multiple feet that made up the intestines.

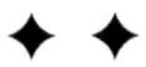

As I came out of the painful mess that was my first round of side-effects, I started to notice my hair showing up more and more on the furniture and blankets, my hair was always falling out or filling my hair appliances. This seemed to be even more. I had my hair cut from its usual shoulder length to about two inches long. It was a nice cut and my friends and family thought it looked good, but I was recovering from surgery at the time and didn't have time to take care of the style, but these little two inch strands were showing up everywhere. I knew the time was coming for all of it to come out. I was scared so I waited for Chris to get home. Putting a drain screen in the kitchen sink drain, I bent over to wash my hair in the sink. As I washed I could feel the hair sticking to my hands and I didn't want to look. I kept my eyes closed and kept rinsing the hair off my hands and the soap out of my hair. After about five minutes I stopped, reached for a towel to wrap around my head, shut off the water, and turned to walk away before I opened my eyes again. I asked Chris to clean out the screen. He did and I asked:

"Is it bad?"

"There's a lot."

"I'm afraid to look."

I had this vision of chunks of hair still stuck on my head in spots that I would have to shave. I walked into the bedroom and removed the towel, it wasn't as bad as I thought. The hair had thinned but was still there. I felt better.

Over the next few days, the rest of it would come out slowly. I lost about 75% of my hair. I also lost about 75% of my eyebrows and eyelashes. The hair on my legs and under my arms stopped growing, as well as my entire pubic area (careful what you wish for when you say you hate to shave). I think the loss of my eyelashes and eyebrows were the worst loss suffered. I had never used eyebrow pencils and although my eyelashes weren't lush, they were mine. Replacing these two things or covering up their absence from my body was going to be a way bigger issue than the "wigs" I thought I was going to need.

Of all the side effects, the hair loss was the easiest to take and the easiest to handle on an ongoing basis. As people, we are very attached to the physical self and how we present to other people. I watched a homeless man once, as someone dropped $5 into his cup wipe his dirty hand on his dirty clothes and extend it to shake the stranger's hand and thank him. It's that moment right there that sums up the loss of your physical hair. We are always trying with whatever we are given to put our best foot forward. The act of the attempt to make sure his hand was in his own opinion clean enough to shake another person's hand is his view of his physical self. Hair works like that. There is a reason that corporations- with an 'S'- make billions of dollars on hair products as well as of all types hair enhancements, ornaments, and restoration products. You add makeup for the eyelashes and eyebrows; you know we are a world of people who live for these types of things and how well we present our physical self to others.

I ran out like every other woman does, to a wig store. Chris's mom bought me a wig, and several pairs of eyelashes, as well as pencils and powder to draw on eyebrows. I made sure I was ready and I wore the wigs… at first.

Then there were the taste buds. Mine were never right after the surgery. It bummed me out. My dad kept saying that everything tasted bland to him on chemo. I had taste, but it was strange. It seemed like everything I was eating was smothered or cooked with butter on it. I could taste the item in a faint way but this overwhelming taste of butter kept creeping in. It was an annoyance but easy to handle. I also found that I couldn't eat certain things and those things became apparent immediately, making me ill not long after I ate them (and in some rare cases, while I was eating them). Once I had made it through the endless days of nausea and vomiting and my appetite returned, I would try small meals with the family. One of the things I couldn't stomach on chemotherapy was most meats, fish and seafood, and chicken could only be consumed in very limited quantities. I tried things over and over, and certain ones exited my body as soon as I ate them, others made the next day very unpleasant.

I did not know how I was going to make it through six more of this treatment. I also expressed disgust in the fact that I wanted to go back to working full time and thought that after the first treatment I would be able to figure out all that. My thought processes was that once I knew what it was like I could go into work to my boss with a plan on how I was going to handle it. I looked at Chris during one of my vomiting spells and said:

"How the hell am I supposed to be able to go into the office and work like this?"

"Chemo hurts."

~Jan Ansley,
Social media status update – two days into her very first chemotherapy treatment.

CHAPTER FIFTEEN
A REASON TO MOVE FORWARD

In two weeks' time, I had experienced it all. I was amazed that when I came out of the side-effects more than a half-month later that I was feeling pretty good. I still was only six weeks out of surgery but when side effects relating to constipation and vomiting subsided they did so completely.

Post-surgery so many things had happened to my body; food didn't taste right; I couldn't walk or sit like I normally could. I didn't have the stamina I once had. Then there was the part that bothered me emotionally; I felt like my home, family, friends and work were getting away from me. I set out to change that. Every day in our small bungalow I would walk back and forth after The Other left for work. It was thirty-two steps from the front door to the bathroom. Not a lot of room but enough for me. So as the sitcoms and TV shows passed on the TV, I would get up every half hour and walk at least four times back and forth from the front door to the bathroom. It took two more weeks before I could navigate the thirteen steps to the basement where I could then walk back and forth in a straighter path. Our basement was twenty eight feet across, and I figured out that approximately a hundred times from wall-to-wall and back was a mile. I would head down stairs four times a day and do a quarter mile. I was waiting until I felt well enough to actually get back on the treadmill that had been collecting dust in the garage since the surgery.

The more I moved, the easier it got and the better I started to feel. I also made it a point every day to log in to work and do something; and as the days turned into weeks, work once again became my priority. I started making dinners again. The Little One came back from his mom's house right after Labor Day and started Junior High. I used to sit with him while he was in grade school and watch him do his homework. Now he was old enough to sit at the kitchen table by himself and knock it out. I kept my fingers crossed that me not ruling homework with an iron fist wouldn't result in his all A's tanking, but I was still within earshot if he needed to ask a question. Because of budget cuts, they had cancelled bus service. It was 1.87 miles from address to address, and the Little One was only twelve going into 8th grade, so there was the matter of getting him to and from school. Walking home, we didn't see as an issue because he had friends to walk with and it would be light out, but in the morning, that wasn't going to work. It was still dark and the new parade of derelicts in our neighborhood caused by the housing bubble and the newly created rental homes had me a bit nervous. Then, there was the matter of Michigan winters. Could he really walk two miles in 3-6 inches of snow? I did a mile as a middle school kid but that was the 1970's, and I had been walking to school since kindergarten. The school was partly accommodating before school, opening up two hours early so that the kids could be dropped off on the parent's way to work. It was the afterschool on bad weather days that could be an issue. Chris worked more than an hour from our house which had him leaving at 6:40am and usually not home before 5:30. I knew I could get him there on the days I felt good, but what about those two weeks a month with chemo—how was I going to work that out?

The biggest suggestion was from other parents for ride sharing, only that wouldn't work. Chris could only do the morning drop off, so that meant you were asking another child to get up ninety minutes early for school, and we didn't have a parent close by whose child actually went to school every day like ours did. I watched when I was out of work and saw the kids that were home all the time on school days. When I would ask The Little One there was always some excuse:

"His mom overslept."

"She had to go to the Ortho."

"Their grandma was visiting."

Nothing at all that I would let ours stay home for.

The stress of the situation mounted on me as the start of school came, I was franticly wondering what I could possibly do. I knew there was no way I could get him being so sick. We finally figured out that physically I would only have to drive on three sick days. He took piano and his grandmother picked him up on Tuesdays, and his mom had volunteered to help if she could and I thought we could ask her to pick him up on Fridays a few hours earlier. This settled my worry a little; I thought three days I could manage, already putting out of my head the last words from the round of chemotherapy I had been through "never again." Not to mention the fact that I couldn't figure out how I was going to drive while in a chemo coma or worse yet… while vomiting.

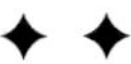

That wasn't the only stress. I had to visit the hospital twice that September-once at the beginning of the third week and then a couple days before my next chemo. They would draw blood and do a CA125. I hadn't thought about that test at all since I was first given my numbers pre-surgery, and as I went back to the hospital to get blood drawn, I didn't think much about it other than I was irritated that they couldn't draw blood from my port. When I had it installed they told me they could, and yet as I was now having blood drawn in what seemed like an every-other-week basis, I was starting to get annoyed. My arms were bruised up and not every girl who worked there when I said 'butterfly needle' listen to me causing unnecessary pain and bruising.

It cost me three dollars every trip to the hospital plus the gas of the twenty mile round trip at four dollars a gallon. I had no other choice. They 'highly recommended' that I have the blood work done there, so they would have it in the computer to check on and evaluate before the next chemo. There were no 'free' lots within walking distance and since I was not at 100% post-surgery I don't know if I could have walked even if I wanted to. As it was from the hospital lot, I had to walk about a half a mile to get to the lab. Money was becoming a huge issue. I was put on part-time and desperate to get back to full-time. My company was paying me well to be a part-timer and let me work from home, but as we had just come back in line with our finances after that long layoff, I wasn't ready to go back to that. I was monitoring every penny. It helped that we couldn't go anywhere for weeks and that I really wasn't eating much. In addition, the Little One had been with his mom all summer.

My own frugality also assisted. During my surgery, I had my girlfriend come by and water my pots of flowers, but I discontinued watering the grass and the perennials. We were having a wetter than normal spring and summer, and I thought, they'll come back if I let it go. I managed with these things to knock much out of our budget and keep up on the important things. Around mid-September, the medical bills started rolling in. I was floored that even with insurance, there were many things that weren't covered, or only partially covered. Then, there were co-pays, co-insurance, deductibles and other expenses not covered at all. My pile of medical bills got bigger as the weeks went on, as my paycheck got smaller and smaller. I kept much of this to myself for a short while.

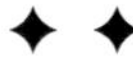

My life with my stepson was very important to me. It was coming up on our fifth year of our co-parenting arrangement with his mom. We each had him fifty percent of the time in large blocks–us during the school year and her during weekends and all vacation time from school. It worked out well for both of our schedules, and when he came back after spending the summer with his mom it was going to fall to me to tell him what had happened while he was gone. He was expecting to come back to us having been married over the summer. Instead, I had to deliver bad news. I knew I didn't want anyone else to do it because I had a way of talking to The Little One where he understood what was being said. I had watched time and time again as other people talked to him, including his own father where I knew he was checking- out, glazing-over and not understanding.

I started the conversation by explaining all that had happened in terms that I thought were appropriate for a twelve-year-old. However, I didn't sugar coat anything. The doctors had told me there was a twenty percent chance that the chemotherapy wouldn't work, and if it didn't it would mean my death. When I finished telling him, I asked if he had any questions. Now, we had talked to him about cancer previous to my conversation, but it obviously didn't go where I needed it to. He knew about my dad's terminal cancer, and he also knew about our friends Brian and Danielle's son Garrett. When Hunter was much younger he played with Garrett often, and we had explained leukemia to him. Yet, his first question on this fall day was:

"Can I catch it?"

I patiently explained why he couldn't and because we weren't related by blood he couldn't even inherit a 'cancer gene' from me. He asked how sick I was going to be and how this was all going to affect his video game time. I was relieved to see that he was thinking about himself like I would expect a pre-teen to act. It made me feel like I had done a good job explaining all this. Then, he asked:

"When will you know if you are in the twenty or eighty percent?"

It was a damn good question and one that I never thought to ask the doctor. I had assumed when he told me that I would be dealing with the nurses and if I had to see him then it was bad news that meant I was doing well, and since they didn't call or even ask how I was doing—beyond me calling the office and asking for help with the side effects—I assumed I was doing well.

I answered him honestly.

"You know, I'm not really sure, but that is a question I will ask as soon as I go for my next chemo."

I asked if there was anything else on his mind, and the words ring in my ears to this day. Now when it comes to this Little One, I have always felt a connection. His personality is so happy. He reminds me of me when I was young. I wanted everyone to be happy and never yell or have problems. I understood those feelings–having had them myself growing up. I tried when things didn't go perfectly to help him work through it, explaining what I didn't understand as a child. Nobody ever explained to me that it isn't all perfect or why it couldn't be, and we have to learn in life to cope with that. I still had to admire him for always wanting to be happy. Knowing that about this Little One, I was still surprised, touched, and emotionally moved to action when the next statement came out of his mouth:

"This will work 'cause you can't leave me here with these people."

He said it so matter of fact, in a way that said to me- *Kim you always fix everything, fix this-* I knew what he meant by these people. I also knew that this was a young boy almost a teenager who still had a mother and father and extended family who loved him dearly and he would be fine if I wasn't in the picture. Yet, it pulled at me. Except for Chris, he was the first to tell me why he needed me around.

Until that point, everyone had said to me:

"You're the strongest person I know. If anyone can beat this you can."

"You are young. You will fight the good fight and be able to beat this."

"If anyone can, you can. Your personality and perseverance will get you through."

Nobody except for Chris had told me why they actually needed me here.

It gave me the reason I needed to take on chemotherapy head first, the piece to the puzzle I had been missing.

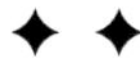

As the fourth Friday in my rotation approached for my second chemotherapy round, I was surprised at how calm I was. I wasn't thinking about blood work and what 'the numbers' meant at this point, and I wasn't thinking about all the things that happened after I received the first dose of chemotherapy. I had blocked most of it out from my memory. The pain, the sickness, it was all like it had never happened. I told myself that all those side-effects were from being just out of surgery. That it wasn't going to be that bad this time.

Over the month, I had reached out on the social media sites to a few people who had come forward upon learning of my diagnosis to tell me they had cancer. They were all in various stages of remission, some had several go rounds with chemo, others only had to go through it once. I asked over the course of the month many questions regarding side-effects. Most of their answers were fairly uniform about how they fought and wouldn't let it get the best of them. They went to work while on chemo, and participated in their daily lives. All my questions were met with positive reinforcement; they gave me their phone numbers and sent texts to check on me. There was a fourth person who was more involved in my life, having been through not one but two cancers and several go rounds with treatment. She was a bit more honest in helping me with side-effect information and how to treat it. She would give specifics on what to eat and how to try and control things. She knew more about the medicines. Not because she had been through it, but her close family members had been through the big fight with cancer. Yet, even with all these people at my disposal, I felt like I wasn't being told something, or that I wasn't asking the question the correct way to get the answer I thought I might need. This big blank kept coming up in my brain when it came to information on chemotherapy as I read and reread all the cancer sites. They all seemed to say the same thing over and over.

It was all so clean and pristine-almost sanitary. Everything worded in a neat little package for the general public to get information... you know, "when you're unfortunate enough to become sick" kind of a one- size-fits-all. All displayed on colorful pages with orderly tabs for easy reference.

I bought right into it, and headed for chemotherapy number two. The medicines were the same, and the time spent there was the same. This time I wrote down daily what had happened to me and told the nurse that administered my chemo. She seemed a bit more on top of things then the girl I had had the month before. I had seen her in there four weeks ago working her butt off. However, I had no personal contact with her. She seemed more knowledgeable or at least more willing to share her knowledge. When I told her everything that had happened she sent for the oncology nurse. This time, instead of the crab-ass who didn't listen, a different girl came in and said:

"I heard you have some questions and concerns." She spoke with a more sympathetic tone.

I relayed what had taken place and the timing. She patiently explained the importance of eating correctly and drinking water, and I explained I would do that if I could get off the bathroom floor. She said to make sure I took both anti-nausea meds; she prescribed a stool-softener to also take for the first four days, and she gave me another script for the Zofran and Compazine when I told her there was no refill on either. She also wrote me a prescription for Motrin 600 to take for the leg and pain issues. I liked her much more than the first girl, even though her last words were, *"Now make these 'scripts last as long as you can."*

As she left, the room I said to Chris's mom:

"Bullshit, I'll take as many as I need."

"I would too. Why wouldn't you? Don't they understand how sick you get?" Sue had as much distain in her voice as I did.

"I don't think they do."

"Well, you can't be the only one that has ever gotten sick."

"No, I can't."

Sue broached a valid point. However something nagged at me. I couldn't help but think to myself, maybe it was because of the surgery. After all, I had talked to three people who had gone through chemotherapy for multiple rounds and they all seemed to blow off my statements about how sick I was.

We finished up and headed home. I set up myself on the couch as Chris's mom went and got the scripts filled right in the hospital. I wasted no time and took my first Zofran when I walked through the door at home, and set up the calendar on my phone for the next eight days to go off in four hour intervals, reminding me which pill to take, so I wouldn't lose track. I also set a reminder for Sunday morning, afternoon, and early evening about taking Motrin at the first sign of the unrelenting twitching and pains and a morning reminder for the stool softener, just to be safe, an hour after I took the Zofran.

I again didn't sleep for two days. I didn't feel great but things were more bearable. The chemo- coma kicked in right after the steroids wore off, which made me think it was definitely the Compazine causing that particular side-effect. In addition, I was suspecting the steroid of causing that uncomfortable anxious feeling I was experiencing on the first two days. I took every pill on time and forced myself to eat and drink something at the time I took each pill. By day four, I still hadn't taken a shit. My dad called and Chris talked to him, he explained how it was all starting again. After being on a pill form of chemo for months, my dad said to Chris:

"I feel her pain. First you can't go then it's diarrhea for days! Tell her to try this over the counter fiber additive two or three times a day. It gets me going."

When Chris hung up the phone, he went to the store and bought the biggest box of the brand my dad had recommended that he could find. It was in those little packets that you add to water bottles. He thought that would be easy—no measuring. I found a sixteen ounce glass, added the packet to whatever I was drinking and did the same ever morning for the next three days.

So, if you are keeping track, I was now taking two anti-nausea meds, Motrin 600 for pain, a stool softener, and a fiber additive. I was drinking only water with the exception of a juice for breakfast to mix the fiber additive into. I thought I was doing well. I didn't want to get mouth sores on top of everything else–something that I had heard another patient talking about while I was in the rest room at chemotherapy–so I had taken to sucking on ice pops throughout the day and whenever I was awake at night. My diet consisted of nothing nutritious or good for me, mostly because the doctor told me to eat what I could keep down, and my well-meaning online buddies had mentioned not to eat anything that I love because I might hate it after chemo. I was eating things that I would never eat if I wasn't under the influence of chemotherapy medications: glazed donuts, taco's from a fast food place, plain mashed potatoes and noodles. Not a fruit or a vegetable in the bunch. Now, I was never the best eater, but I tried as I got older to eat better. Every book by a cancer patient highly recommended changing your diet to a high in vegetable low in sugar and sodium type thing. I thought that meant after chemo stopped. I wasn't taking in any nutrients now, and it didn't dawn on me that it was a bad thing.... because a doctor said "don't worry about it, eat what you can keep down." He never elaborated on what that meant.

All words, all phrases mean different things to different people. I would write about it in my blog and counsel many people about 'intent' when using email, text, or social media. These are all really wonderful things, and yet, unless you are skilled, it is difficult to get a point across. Not everything is black and white. Sometimes you must push for more information. When speaking, it is important to realize that not everyone knows all the details you do.

For example, if I were teaching you how to be a bartender, and you asked me:

"What goes in a Manhattan?"

Now I know, I am the teacher, and I know there are tweaks to all bartending rules because I know how to bartend, but if I say to you:

"Sweet vermouth and whiskey with a cherry garnish."

I would not be wrong, and you would know how to make a Manhattan. You would fumble through getting the details correct as you became more experienced.

However, what I really should have said, so you have the complete picture is,

"Sweet vermouth and whiskey-except for Southern Comfort. It gets dry vermouth because it is a sweet whiskey, unless the customer asks for it sweet, then add sweet vermouth. Oh and one other thing – if the customer asks for their Manhattan perfect, you use both sweet and dry vermouth with the whiskey."

It is my opinion that my doctor was at best vague with his statement about food without even asking if I needed counsel and perhaps suggesting a website or nutritionist. Once again, only being two treatments into it, I didn't think about it in any way or consider asking any questions when I had seen the doctor over six weeks ago. I also found his staff to be unhelpful and just as vague.

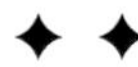

Sunday night the leg pains began and I took the Motrin. It produced some relief, but the pain was still present and more than noticeable. I lay on the bed in the propped up position and asked Chris to rub my legs, hoping it would help. He did and talked softly while he massaged them. The physical act of pressure on my joints and muscles seemed to take away the pain for the moment he pressed on them, but as his fingers moved up and down my legs, I noticed that the moment the pressure was removed the pain came back. I asked repeatedly over the next several hours for the massage—just to grab the moments of relief in-between.

I was still in a chemo-coma later into the week. My stomach was upset but I wasn't vomiting. I also wasn't pooping. It was late on Thursday night, when I reached for my pills as the reminder ding on my phone went off, that it happened again. I made myself a bowl of cereal, and it all came back up. I was devastated. I thought for sure I had made it through. After all, it had been six days. I only vomited that one time, mostly because I didn't really eat again after that, but the pill I had taken was the Compazine (which I ended up vomiting up), and by the time the Zofran came back around I noticed the chemo-coma was gone. Friday and Saturday, I took the Zofran and no Compazine with my last pill on Saturday before bed. On Sunday morning, the bowel pain began again and the rock hard stools that I had to dig out.

Frustrated on Sunday night(ten days after chemo), I googled differently.

Instead of googling things proceeded by the word "Cancer," I googled things like 'constipation,' 'painful bowel movements,' and 'hard stools.' I came up with answers relating to things I know I didn't have: 'irritable bowel syndrome,' 'diverticulitis,' and 'Crohn's.' I had almost given up when I decided to type: 'painful bowel movements after a hysterectomy.' Up popped two sites: one with information on the hysterectomy and one with information plus a section with a chat room with questions and answers from actual people. I looked into the thread on the one site's chat room and there laid before me was one anonymous post after another about the pain women suffered after the hysterectomy with bowel movements. Nobody had an answer but they shared: how they would shred through a roll of toilet paper, several broke things in the bathroom like doors off cabinets and towel bars in an effort to control the severe pain. As I read over and over again about the duration, it matched mine after the surgery, but as I read on, I couldn't find anyone who then went on to chemotherapy treatment and had the same pain. I spent two days on that site. There were thousands of posts. All the same relating to the severity of the pain in restarting the bowels, and it all sounded like mine.

I was thinking that maybe I was looking at this all wrong, and perhaps after all this, it was the hysterectomy causing the issue, not the chemotherapy. After all, the people I had talked to with cancer didn't seem as sick as me from what they were telling me.

CHAPTER SIXTEEN
TOUGH LADY, THIS IS AS GOOD AS IT GETS

The month I spent between Treatment two and three, I continued the routine I had started. The pain and utter discomfort I spent in Round Two was decreased because I had pills to assist with the side effects at the start, but not by much. It is like the difference between half-full and half-empty glass interpretation; positive and negative. I didn't spend as much time vomiting profusely, but I did vomit several times in the last days. The leg pains weren't as intense but they were there noticeable and disruptive. The problems in the potty never changed even with a stool softener and extra fiber; in fact they were worse with the added fiber—adding a whole other layer of cramping.

I researched more that month. Removing the word cancer from my side-effect questions and slowly finding obscure sites and blogs, there seemed to be this whole underbelly to the glitz and glamour. The more I read from actual people the more annoyed I became. About half way through that month I re-emailed the people I had originally emailed and asked very specific questions, not just general questions about side-effects. All three online still gave me vague answers, more along the lines of '*yes there were rough patches, but be strong; you'll get through them, and then everything will be fine. I'm here for you.*' The fourth, the girl I actually had contact with, was more forthright and answered questions directly. I was surprised by both. As I read on in different threads and comment forums, a whole new picture started to come together about side-effects and dealing with them. The exact same thing that was happening to me; the human body and its brain has tremendous abilities. One of those abilities is the power of protection over its own self. In other words, as I stated before, once the side-effects were over, the body forgets how it feels and how horrific the ordeal was. It is this protection, I truly believe, that was *masking* things in the cancer world. As I read over and over when a question was asked about some horrific side-effect being posted by a caretaker of a patient searching for help as it happened, there was a stream of comments and posts about, *'yes, it happened to me, but I got through it and so will you or your loved one.'*

I found this to be incredibly unacceptable. I believe the statements were only meant with true compassion and only the best of intentions as a means to encourage people through horrific circumstances and side-effects. With that said, the statements did nothing to help assist people in knowing anything about these monstrous happenings. Many people gave no real clue as to what to do about them, or how to handle side-effects in any way, shape or form.

I was also dumb founded with all the things I read. All the information I had watched on TV, and my doctors and nurses... No one thought it was important to explain what chemotherapy is going to actually 'feel' like, or the fact that there would be *two* sets of side-effects going on at the same time–one from the surgery and one from the chemotherapy. It felt like a big cover up. I sat one night reading, and an offshoot article that caught my eye; a former prisoner was speaking out about his mistreatment in prison. I laughed and thought: *'You're a prisoner'* with my usual sarcasm. As I read the entire article half-heartedly, I realized something, he was making demands, and people were listening to him over things that I thought were ridiculous. Poor me, we don't get internet time; poor me they feed us bad food; poor me, I want. I remembered the prisoners-of-war over in Iraq that the military took 'humiliating' pictures of and then suffered the repercussions of those actions, and I said out loud for the first time:

"That's humiliating? Try chemotherapy! They'll talk!"

"What?" Chris said looking up from his magazine.

"You know, we treat prisoners better than chemotherapy patients."

"You're probably right."

I said no more at that moment, but that thought stayed with me.

Also, that month was the first time I was approached by someone to ask me about cancer. She would be the first of many referred to me by a mutual acquaintance. I received an email stating who she was, how she got my name, and would it be alright since she was just diagnosed if she could ask me some questions when she had them. I agreed but in return asked her a few things, so I could advise her correctly. Was she married? Did she or her husband work full-time and did she have kids? Things nobody ever asked me about. In other words, when chemotherapy hits, do you have someone to assume your daily responsibilities' and take care of you? She said she was a stay-at-home mom with three small children and her husband worked a full and part-time job.

So before she could ask her first question, I sent her a four page word document explaining that her husband needed to cut back on his hours at work immediately following treatment as she would need help taking care of her 2, 3, and 6-year-old for that week following chemo. She was shocked at my candor when I told her to prepare for the worse pain in her life along with other things. She thanked me and started chemo. Three weeks later she emailed me again and told me how when she asked her doctor about the things I had wrote to her about he told her, *"I was an extreme case, and that there was some bad doctoring there, not to worry that everybody's different."* There was that ridiculous terminology again. Every medical professional that I had contact with used it, as well as every cancer patient. *"Well everybody's different but…"* She then went on to tell me about the muscle and joint pain, the extreme nausea and constipation. After listening to her doctor, she didn't bother to ask anyone to help her with the kids, trusting the doctor over me (like she should) and by day four her husband had to call in sick and try to line up people to come to the house over the next few days to assist her. She said she felt like she was back-tracking and could have had her mother or aunt drive in and stay with them for the week if she could have given them some notice.

Then she asked me, "Why do they lie?"

I didn't have an answer for her, and I honestly don't think medical professionals are lying. With that said, I do think they say only what the lawyers tell them they can, a very generic non- threatening, not-so-scary *"everybody's different."*

I was upset that this new virtual person I had met was going through all this without help, but I was also justified in my new confirmation that it wasn't just me who was this sick. Everybody is different –it's a matter of how many times or days you are going to be sick compared to me. Her muscles and joint pain seemed even more severe than mine and it also seemed to last for days and days, and her vomiting was less, but still there. She also came back around after six days. So, we were different. But we were both very, very sick. I questioned a friend of mine more at that point about the level of her illness. She admitted the severity of how sick she was, laying on the living room floor but determined never to miss work and let cancer 'win.'

Now, I had four confirmed very sick people out of the eight people I knew with cancer. I thought it was time to push. I sent one last email to my virtual friends and asked as direct as I could:

"Did you vomit?"

"Did you shit yourself?"

Or *"Did you not poop for more than 5 days?"*

"How severe was your pain?"

"What exactly did your nausea feel like?"

All three responded with very long emails, words that I think they had been holding back for years in two of the cases:

"...I never wanted to think of those moments again. It was the worst time in my life.."

"...I don't know why you wanted to know this Kim, but yes, I would get up and run for the bathroom, shitting myself with every step. It got to where I couldn't leave the house. When I told my doctor, he prescribed a pill. I can't remember the name anymore. I thought he had given me tic-tacs because they didn't work..."

"...By the third round of chemo I asked for sleeping pills and took them every 12 hours. My grandmother watched me. I couldn't stand the pain anymore and choose to sleep through it..."

That was seven. The last person being my father; I didn't know how to go about asking him directly, but I knew I could get info. So, I went where all good daughters go, to my sisters. I asked them and my mom how my dad was doing. I lived the farthest from my parents and over the last few years , I was only seeing them in person less than once a month. I used to see them daily when I lived on their side of town. When it came to my parents, and in particular my dad's cancer, I managed to convince myself that I didn't really need to think about it, avoiding the subject, avoiding visiting, avoiding the consequences of his multiple myeloma. A different picture presented itself. As the conversations went on about the good days and bad days, it was then I knew it was eight out of eight that were very sick with chemo. That the pills they gave you for side-effects, although they made you better than previous years, were nowhere to the level of treating these side-effects as they should be.

...And I didn't like that thought and what it meant when it came to my future in dealing with this cancer within me. Because it said to me: Tough luck lady. This is as good as it gonna get. Everybody's suffering.

CHAPTER SEVENTEEN

COME OUT, COME OUT WHERE EVER YOU ARE

By the time I got through my side-effects on chemo number three, I was a fireball. Not just physically from the hot flashes but in my anger over how sick I was. I gave up trying to tell the nurses in the cancer center and at the doctor's office because they weren't listening or understanding me, and I didn't know how to make myself clearer. Every person that visited me or called I talked about how sick I was, and yet I wasn't sure all of them got it. TMI! TMI! I would hear over and over. Those 'too much information' conversations got me the much needed support from family and friends to keep me moving forward, but I still felt like I needed to keep talking. I set out to find a support group. I was pretty much healed from the surgery at that point, and I was mobile when I wasn't sick from the chemo, which gave me two solid weeks a month of feeling decent. Nowhere near my old self, but about 70% of what I used to be. I looked on-line. I called a few places, but nobody had what I wanted: a group where I could sit and talk about what I was going through with a bunch of other cancer patients. I wanted to know if I could learn anything from them and how they coped. There were groups *'look good, feel good'* being the biggest and most common. When I called the girl told me it was tips on makeup and wigs, but she wasn't sure they would talk about other things. That wasn't going to cut it. I didn't want to stop a conversation to learn about eye shadow. Putting makeup on was the least of my worries. There were dozens of videos on-line with cancer patients showing you things like that. I wanted the nitty-gritty of how other people coped and how their friends and family treated them.

There was no doubt that some of our friends had fallen off

the grid. People who I had previously heard from weekly stopped sending emails or coming by. I was irritated by that but managed to talk through it with Chris and we figured that new people were filling those spots. I also watched as people took complete advantage of the fact that I was sick; to move themselves into better positions in life because of my absence.

These things frustrated me, and left me with only very close friends and my immediate family to vent to, and that was a source that I felt was soon going to be tapped out. I mean you can only listen to somebody whine for so long, and I had spent every moment I was allotted with the people in my life to whine and vent. I checked into a private therapist but at one hundred and twenty dollars an hour that wasn't going to happen. This left me alone with my thoughts and ideas about this whole cancer thing. It also forced me focus on all angles not just the "poor me" side. All by myself.

I rarely wore my wigs anymore, saving them for when I was going to go back to work at the office in January, which I kept telling myself would happen. When you wear the scarf, people know for sure you have cancer. It's a mark on you. As if you were wearing a sandwich board walking up and down a busy street. As I was able to venture out more and more, I started to notice other people's reactions to me. Some would grab their kids and move away quickly, others would stare trying not to get caught, and several older ladies would come over and let me know that they were 'survivors' and give me a brief summary of their cancer which always included type of cancer, number of treatments, and length of survival to date. Then, they would wait for me to let them know the same about me. They would wish me luck, and I would be on my way. I started to be able to pick the wigs out in a crowd, and by the drawn on eyebrows I could tell if I was dealing with a cancer patient. It's always harder with men because so many shave their heads anyways, but that lack of eyebrows and no five o'clock shadow were always a give-away. I started to see more and more people, at the mall, the supermarket and local eateries. In the ten years I had lived in the area I currently live in, I had never seen anyone in a cancer scarf or turban, I wore mine proudly. I wanted people to know. I wanted EVERYONE to know.

It seemed odd that the more I paid attention, the more I realized there were people everywhere I went, everywhere I looked, and even within my own circle who were 'hiding' the fact that they had cancer.

So I started to poke. Just like a nervous repetitive habit such as picking at a flaw on an object till you manage to smooth out the rough spot, I started to see a pattern. A pattern that scared the hell out of me. It made me realize that even though going into this I knew what cancer was; it was becoming increasing clear why I never really understood it. I kept likening it to a major cover-up.

I couldn't understand this rush to 'normal'. The people with cancer were very good at hiding, covering up their illness so nobody knew; all under the disguise that 'cancer won't define me'.

It does define you. It changes your physical self, your emotional self, your money, and the people you share your life with: everything gets touched by it.

These people are correct to a point that you must and need to continue on with your life. There are stories floating around everywhere about people who get married and spend their honeymoon in chemotherapy, finish up a huge art project, or some other labor of love. People who continue running large companies or fulfill their duties some other way; but what I don't understand is that as you do this you should be telling everyone in your path:

"I am sicker than I've ever been and I'm still going to continue on."

I believe there isn't enough loud complaining about this thing known as cancer. It's great that we want to lift up and support everyone, but why can't we let the people on the outside see that we are honoring these cancer survivors because they've been to hell and back, and tell them exactly what that looks like. Instead, we tie pretty, pink ribbons on everybody and wear clever T-shirts. I want to hear someone on a commercial for one of these huge moneymakers say:

"I'm walking for my sister who spent the better part of ten months lying in bed crying over the pain in her joints, missing her boobs, thinking she was ugly. The vomiting has stopped and now we walk."

"I want it to be okay to go to work in a scarf not an itchy wig that you constantly have to monitor to make sure it didn't shift or is sticking out in some weird form and that's why I help."

"I want people to know that I am walking through the store today pushing a shopping cart and that yesterday I was dying on the bathroom floor. That it is a huge accomplishment for me. Now, I am here. I've been to hell and back and I'll never be the same."

"I don't want people to have to lie to keep their jobs. So many people, I was starting to realize, didn't share what was happening for fear of losing their job. So I am here to let everyone know, let us work if we want to and feel we can. Better yet, let's find a cure so we don't have to worry about any of this."

"When you think about all the times in your life you spent angry, upset, annoyed…. What an incredible waste of time."

- Kim Henderly
  So I Age~The Ramblings of A Caffeine Induced Mind
  November 2010

CHAPTER EIGHTEEN
THE PARTY

As the months moved on, my isolation was getting to me. My BFF Charlotte had given birth prematurely a few months before my surgery and I needed to feel normal and sit with her for an afternoon. I missed our 'her and I' time. Charlotte's husband called us 'two peas in a pod.' We were educated, common-sense oriented women with big mouths and not just the types who give you our opinion; we had a high decibel range when we got together. She was very busy with her own life: she traveled for work, had her new son, a home and husband to take care of. Yet she found a weekday afternoon to come by when I was alone. We sat and talked and as the afternoon rolled on, I realized I had nothing to say unless it related to my cancer. I actually said to her toward the end of the afternoon:

"This is all I have to talk about."

But, Charlotte took away something much bigger from that conversation.

It wasn't long after that when she approached me about hosting a party in my honor; my sister Jennifer had also said she wanted to do something to help. Cancer takes a toll on your budget. The cost, even with insurance is great; there are details that you have to pay for like any illness that you don't know about until you go through them. Then, there are the extras that you don't think about that aren't covered by insurance: adult diapers, bandages after the surgery, pads for the bed so you don't destroy your mattress, parking costs at the hospital, utility bills go up because you are home more than before, and your paycheck goes way down because you aren't working full-time anymore. If your caretaker burns through their vacation days and you still need assistance, now they're not being paid. If I would have had breast cancer, there were a bunch of organizations that would have assisted me with money for bills,(both personal and medical), food, housekeeping, the list goes on. But each place I called, each email I sent was denied because I had ovarian cancer, the wrong cancer.

I put Charlotte and Jennifer together, and never a better team had been formed. My organized, down-to-the-minute BFF and my highly motivated and talented, over-extended sister divided the event into sections and ran with it, each enlisting their own family and friends to help. The night turned out to be a wonderful party and all my friends and family were there. Along with our close friends Brian and Danielle, and my other two sisters Michaelene and Paula were all spending much of their own personal time and money on the party.

I got to dance for the first time in months with Chris, laugh and tell my story to people I hadn't seen since the surgery. It was an important moment in my life, and the people that came to that party, which had been named Project O by Jennifer, meant the world to me. I thanked everyone that evening with the following speech, which I am happy to say I didn't choke up on until the very end. I posted the speech on my blog the next day.....

I have always been the older sister, someone's boss, the band's manager. I am the one that buys the tickets and knocks back vodka gimlets and beer at these types of things. So to be in a position where I have to ask for help for myself is ...difficult...and without getting on a soap box and preaching about the state of the world's greatest healthcare system and how ridiculously expensive it is...

When you are social people like Chris and myself, a lot of things can slow you down, and take away your fun temporarily – work, family, getting bronchitis.

The day the doctor walked into my hospital room following surgery, he acted just as I would want a doctor to act– he shot straight from the hip. Made no excuses, gave me my diagnosis and what could be done. He let me know what my chances of survival are.

His visit was followed by a hospital worker, who sat on my bed looked me in the eye and said, "I've lain where you are. You get one day. One day to feel sorry for yourself, then cancer becomes your full-time job."

Now, anyone who has worked with me knows that statement was probably the best thing she could have said. I took my day. I had Chris text everyone and said no visitors. And, I got ready to spend the next twenty-four hours feeling sorry for myself.

I started where most people do. What could I have done differently? I thought about my life and everyone who had touched it. I started to smile again. You see, what kept popping in my head where all the things that made me laugh. It was the happiness that others had brought to me that was coming through loud and clear. Gone were the memories that upset me. When you think about all the times in your life you spent angry, upset, annoyed…what an incredible waste of time!

I didn't sleep those twenty-four hours. Instead, I lay in that hospital bed, and, listening to my roommate eat all night, I played over and over the things that had touched me. My sisters make fun of me because of my idyllic memory. Yet, it was all I had. I realized something in that hospital bed.

That social Kim and Chris were the only thing that was going to get me through this.

In the months that have followed that surgery and diagnosis:

Friends both old and new came from everywhere: texting, emailing, sending cards and gifts, calling, and stopping by. They made me laugh when I got angry over side-effects. They gave me encouragement when I was scared of the next step. They showed up at my door week after week, day after day and told me I looked great, even without hair, eyebrows and eyelashes.

I compared side-effects with those in my life who are also fighting this horrible battle. And people listened when I only had one topic of conversation. They understood that social events would now take place in living-rooms and not the bars… And they somehow knew that this is what I needed.

So thank you, for bringing me lunch, for sitting on the couch, for emailing me, for asking if I need anything, for being my friends and not leaving me behind in the dust while you continued a life without me.

Thank you for not giving up on me.

Thank you for being here tonight. You have helped Social Kim and Chris more than you will ever know.

It was the best night, and even though the conversation revolved around cancer for the majority of the night, I felt more like my old self than I had since June 30th.

CHAPTER NINETEEN
IT'S ALL ABOUT THE NUMBER

I lucked out when it came to the holidays. Chemo number five hit on Friday December 3rd, and there were five Fridays that year, my next chemo would be Friday, December 31st leaving my birthday and Christmas open for me to celebrate with family and friends. Since the cancer center was going to be closed on New Year's Eve, they pushed my sixth treatment to January 3, 2011.

As I sat down for my fifth chemo with my friend Danielle accompanying me, I asked first thing for the numbers. For me, like most patients, they had become by that time: an obsession. At my second session, the nurse I liked printed them out for me for all my blood draws. It was the first time I realized that I could get that information without talking to the doctor, and by the time treatment number four came up I was able to explain to my sister Michaelene, as she sat there with me what some of the numbers meant. I always glanced first down the high/low column–which was marked by an asterisk if a number was out of line. If the asterisk was there, I'd glance over to see the H or L signifying if the number was high or low out of normal parameters. Low came up quite a bit and I asked the nurse about it, but she said if it was bad the doctor would contact me. Nobody contacted me, so I didn't worry.

The CA125, out of all the numbers, was the biggie and I always wanted to see it in writing. I had taken to calling the doctor's office and asking for the number the day after my lab work so I knew almost a week before chemo. On that December morning, I knew my number already and was so positive that I was close to the end of my nightmare.

When the numbers hit ninety-six at the start of chemo number five, I told Danielle that hopefully I could really knock this out before number six and maybe wouldn't need the last treatment. All my drops had been around a hundred points. However, I learned after the fact, the lower the number the slower it falls. There is less cancer so, small drops in what *is* eliminated in the body. I was devastated when I called after that fifth treatment, and I had only dropped to fifty-two. I was beginning to think that it wouldn't work. The numbers hardly moved at all compared to the other times. I dreaded that last treatment. The doctor had said if the number doesn't get under thirty-five he might have to hit me with two more. I didn't think I could take two more times of all these side effects. As it was, I was barely making it through and what gave me more strength was the fact that I could see the light at the end of the tunnel. My CA125 looked like this through treatments:

Pre-surgery: 1442
Going into Chemo 1: 596
Going into Chemo 2: 384
Going into Chemo 3: 282
Going into Chemo 4: 188
Going into Chemo 5: 96
Going into Chemo 6: 52

To get through the days, I remembered when I had watched the Gilda Radner movie about her life many years ago. She had put post-it notes on her mirror, ripping them off as she went through treatment. My Aunt Toni, when I had surgery, sent a wonderful little get-well present. Among the items in the gift bag, there was a small cube notepad with cute shoes drawn in black down the sides. I took the pad when chemo started, and wrote the numbers backwards on each sheet starting at 141; it was the number of days from first chemo to last. I ripped the sheets off daily, watching the number go down helped. I tried to think of those days in terms of 'vacation.' You know you start a vacation and think in your head "wow, seven wonderful days' and as they click off and it's your Wednesday of the vacation week, you think, *"Hell, I've still got half a week,"* and on the last you say, *"this week went by so fast."* That's how I tried to approach the numbers. When I dropped out of triple digits, I thought, *"remember when I was way over a hundred"* and nothing was sweeter than to be down under ten. The best pulls were the days after chemo. Since I was sick for so many by the time I got back to the fridge (where I had secured the pad of paper with magnets), I would be able to pull several sheets. I loved watching that number drop.

My sixth round of chemo The Other took me. I had heard that they made a big deal when you finished. People with cancer had told me about 'ringing the bell.' I wanted to have people make a big deal over me, however that didn't happen. It was as busy as ever and the girls were as nice, but I left with no fanfare and when I said I think this might be my last I was told:

"Hopefully. Wait for the numbers, and hope you are done."

That's it? I thought to myself. At least I had Chris here to be happy for me. As I lay in bed, getting sick again on that round, I kept praying that this was the last one and I would be done. I didn't want to jump the gun with work, but I needed to get back to fulltime and resume my life. I started to play how things were going to be different with me once I got through this last one. All the books I had read about people who had made it through, they had all changed their diet and exercise routines to help continue a healthy overall lifestyle. I was planning on doing that also. More vegetables, less fast food, exercise, I started to map out a plan, remembering all the things I had read and doing research for cancer-fighting foods.

My doctor's appointment wouldn't be until the first week in February. This made me wonder. They had to do two blood draws and a CT scan was ordered. As I sat in that sixth chemo, the office girl came by as usual and handed me a calendar. I looked down at it, and saw the blood draws and CT scan listed. Again I had to ask the question.

"Where do I go for this CAT Scan?"

"Across the street at the imaging center. You have to show up ninety minutes early and you can't eat for four hours before you show up"

"This means I have to be there by 3:30? For a 5:00 appointment?" I was upset; I knew that meant leaving work early, even though I would be going back.

"Don't they have a 5:30 or 6:00 appointment?" I asked

"They used to, but not anymore. I don't know why, but I gave you the last one in the day they had. Maybe if you call there, they will give you the contrast to drink and then you won't have to show up early," she suggested

After she left, the nurse, whom I had come to depend on for information, stuck her head in the room:

"Does that calendar have a port flush on it?" she asked.

I liked this nurse. She tried to be honest with me about me questions and gave me information that sometimes I didn't even know I needed. We talked about some personal stuff, and I felt like she had my back in the hospital. It's the kind of feeling I thought I should have gotten from my doctor-assigned oncology nurse.

"No it doesn't. What's that?" I replied.

"Every four or five weeks, you need to come back here and get this port flushed out. You can keep them in a long time, but they have to be cleaned." She went on, in the way she had, like no one else did in the hospital. She told a story or gave an example. *"We have this one lady. She's been in remission seven years and still comes her every four weeks without fail. She says she feels like if she takes out the port it will jinx her and the cancer will come back."* I felt like she was telling me, no matter what they say don't remove the port.

Like I had mentioned, I felt like doctors and nurses were controlled by lawyers, not divulging anything that could get them sued. This girl, because of the connection we had formed, was in her own way giving me some advice. As I looked down at the calendar and realized it was five weeks until I saw the doctor, I couldn't help but wonder once again, why my assigned oncology nurse hadn't told me about getting a port flush?

"So how do I go about doing this? I really can't take a day off work to come here. I know you close at 4:00, can I make a 4:00 appointment?" I asked her. I was thinking, *"Great, leave early for CT scan, leave early for port flush. How the hell are you supposed to be able to maintain a job?"*

"Don't worry. It doesn't take long. I'll make you an appointment and you can come on your lunch. Let me make that for you now and print you another calendar. Four weeks from today good?"

She assigned me an 11:30 time four weeks away, and I added it to the calendar. This meant four separate trips back to the hospital before I even talked to the doctor again. I was holding out that since there was no call for me to come in during these six treatments that things were going as he had planned. At the start of chemo number six, my CA125 was down to fifty-two. A drop from being in the nineties but not the below the thirty-five I had hoped for. The nurse I had come to like, when I had expressed the wish that it would drop me below thirty-five and not need the sixth treatment, had said:

"I think I would take it anyways just too kinda give it that last push to totally be out."

I was thinking, *no way! I wanted to go back to work!* I was driving myself crazy sitting at home only working part-time, and we were getting desperate for the income. The insurance would reset it's self on January 1st, 2011 and that meant a whole new round of co-pays, co-insurance and the like.

I had already requested a full-time start date of January 10 and was pushed back by work to the last week of the month. That was another month's salary lost. I was so close to this nightmare being over, and I wanted my life back to where it was. I started planning. I wanted to spend my weekends traveling with My Other and I couldn't wait until it was me, him, and the Little One again hanging out having fun, just us or with friends, I didn't care. I just wanted my old life: pre-cancer, pre-being sick. I wanted to work on our house and fix up the kitchen and bathroom, maybe do a little redecorating. I hadn't spent enough time with The Little One and pushing him in school like I thought I should.

Most of all, I wanted my energy back. The thing that let me go, go, go for more than fourteen hours a day. I knew I wasn't going to waste a minute of my life. I was going to go out and do even more than before.

CHAPTER TWENTY
CAN I BREATH NOW?

I had dealt with so much over the past several months that when I called the doctor's office on January 28, 2011 I knew everything was going to be okay. I needed it to be okay. I hadn't let one negative thought into my head. No what-if's, no just-in-case, I will have a plan B. Nope, I felt like everything was going to be good.

Coming out of my sixth chemotherapy treatment, I felt good; better than I ever had. I started to shop differently, more vegetables and fruits, nothing processed. I tried not to microwave anything I ate and watched the chemicals I was using around the house. I started exercising again but found it very hard to even get ten minutes in. I pushed myself—starting with simple stretches from an old Jane Fonda VHS I had. It was the middle of one of our harsher winters in Michigan, bitter cold and lots of snow. I started shoveling more but found that where I once could knock out our front driveway and sidewalks, including the packed ice the snow plow leaves behind, I could now only shovel for about five minutes and then I had to come in and rest. I depended on The Little One to carry the majority of the load where once we both were out there. Now it was mostly him with me doing the porch and steps only.

I hid in the ladies room at work and dialed the doctor's office. The girl who ran the office picked up the phone as usual, and as happy as I could sound with my heart pounding in my ears I identified myself and asked the question"

"Can I get the results of my CA125?"

"Sure, Kim, just a sec while I pull it up. Umm..." A wonderful happiness came to her always professional voice *"Twenty-six!!!"*

I felt every nerve in my body release from its tensed state that had been my way of life since June 30, 2010. *"So I can breathe now?"* I said it as a light-hearted statement and because I didn't know what else to say.

"Yes you can. Congratulations!"

I thanked her for the info and said I'd see her at my next appointment and hung up.

I didn't know what to do with myself. My prayers had been answered, and I was in the very lucky eighty percent that make it. I stopped myself, remembering there were twenty percent who didn't make it. I felt so humbled at that moment. I didn't know why I was in the positive percentile, but I knew whatever I had been put on this earth to do, I had not yet accomplished it. I was spared, and I knew I wasn't going to waste a moment of this extra time I had been given.

I said a prayer for all of those who didn't make it when fighting ovarian cancer and thanked God over and over for giving me this second chance, and what did I do next… went back to my desk and continued working. Oh, I spent much of that day emailing people to tell them. But I got all my work done, and knew I wanted to push myself harder in this growing company. I was going to do so much!

I spun my chair around to look at the snow outside the window at work. My cube had been moved when I was working from home from one side of the office to the other. Mostly so the owner could talk to me easier, and I had been assigned some new and exciting tasks. Yet, I had turned my back once again as before, to the window. I liked having the window right by me, but I felt facing it caused daydreaming at work and that's not what I was about. When at work, I was about work. I used what I considered to be my break-time to converse on a personal level with my coworkers, so additional staring out the window would not be tolerated by me and my long-held, self-imposed work ethic. Yet, looking out the window, I couldn't help but remember on that day what Teri, another cancer survivor friend, had told me. She said that everything is more vibrant; the little things that used to drive you crazy, not so important. As I looked out, I saw the sun's effects on the snow, crystallizing the top layer; it sparkled and the sun never looked brighter. Instead of thinking how much the ride in the new snow was going to suck on the way home, I thought about how pretty it was and that I was glad to be able to say I had a full-time job to drive home from. I had been telling friends over the last few months that I seemed to have developed a 'whatever' gene. Things that I couldn't control used to upset me. I worried about everything from whether or not the alarm would go off in the morning to would I have a good night's sleep at the end of the day. The old Kim would obsess over details and things that needed to be done. Yet, this new Kim was glad to be here and felt like she needed to share this new outlook.

I had blogged since 2006 and used the format to express my view on any detail that hit me, and I felt I needed to share. I started to be more selective about what I put out there, leaning towards the positive side instead of being so negative with my take on things.

I turned back to my desk and started working again... *I need to change the layout, so I can look outside more often*, I thought to myself.

I'll add that to the new 'To Do List'.

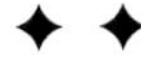

My doctor's appointment was coming up on Tuesday, and the Friday before was the 28th, the day I had called for my CA125 results. It was also the day of my CT Scan. I headed out of work ten minutes before I was supposed to be there, not wanting to leave even a minute early from my recently-returned-to-full-time position. I walked into the imaging center and not only was there not a chair available in this fifty plus seat waiting room, some of the other patients were also standing around outside in the lobby waiting. The room smelled of body odor and that stuffy musty smell rooms get when the heat is too high and the room is too small for all the people. Winter in Michigan requires a heavy coat, and usually by January, those dry-clean-only coats have been worn since the beginning of November and are in desperate need of a good cleaning. I went up to the desk, having left my wig in the car and placed my cancer scarf on. It seemed that it would be obvious to anyone working there why I was there.

I hadn't eaten since noon and with my 'every two hour' rule for eating still in effect, I was feeling the effects of not eating with my nausea level rising by the minute. I signed in, handed over, my insurance info, id and was handed a clip board. I railed through the same questions I had been asked hundreds of times(and more than a dozen time in this very hospital). This time adding ovarian cancer, it's treatment and the surgery from a few months ago. When I handed in the clip board, I was told to wait at the desk. The girl disappeared into a side room and re-emerged with a 32oz Styrofoam cup with a lid and a straw. She instructed me,

"Drink this as quickly as you can. When you are done, bring the cup back to the desk and someone will write down the time. You have to wait exactly one hour, and then they will take you back for your scan."

"Is it alright if I sit in the hall? People are coughing and because of the chemo I don't want to catch anything."

"Yes. They call out in the lobby too."

With that, I headed to the lobby, sat down, and started to drink. It tasted like warm water and I was relieved that it didn't have some weird taste. I was hungry and thirsty and it took less than two minutes for me to drink down the liquid. I walked back to the desk and said I was done.

"Wow, we haven't even put your info into the computer yet." I glanced to see that my clipboard was still sitting on the lower counter. The girl behind the desk went to get a file folder and added a form to it. She noted the time and said someone would call me in an hour. I headed back to the lobby area and called The Other. He was having his own problems; wanting to be there for the scan, he was having trouble negotiating traffic in the newly fallen snow. What is normally an hour drive was going to take a lot longer. I was bummed that he wasn't there to keep me calm, but we talked on the phone as he drove. The hour time slot arrived, and he still hadn't arrived. I decided to hang up to listen for the girl to call my name. At an hour and ten minutes, I walked up to the desk. Now angry because it was past the hour marker and I wanted the test to go well, and because I needed to pee badly. The irritation showed in my voice as I approached the counter:

"Um, excuse me. I was told someone would call me in an hour, it's an hour and ten minutes now. What's going on?"

"Just a little longer," the polite girl behind the counter said.

I raised my voice, so all six girls could hear, mostly because I didn't know which one was in charge, but I had had it with being ignored by hospital personnel. I was forced to leave work a half hour early, and yet they were behind! I wasn't going to let this go this time around.

"Yeah, you told me one hour. Now is this going to mess up the test? And why didn't you call me and have me come a half hour later if you were behind? Is my time not important also?"

I almost laughed when one woman stepped forward and said as a response:

"We used to be open later, but nobody was in here."

I turned and looked at the full waiting room and then turned back to her,

"Well, that doesn't seem to be a problem today. Now you made me leave work to be here. The least you could do is see me on time, and by the way, we're going on an hour an twenty minutes of thirty-two ounces of fluid in a forty-eight-year-old woman. Get this test done before I pee my pants!"

"It will only be a few more minutes."

I took an open seat directly across from the desk; I didn't want them to forget about me. That few minutes turned out to be another fifteen minutes. Unfortunately Chris walked in right after the Radiologist Tech came out to get me, and they wouldn't let him back. I'm sure my punishment for being so vocal.

When the tech called my name and we headed back, she asked how I was doing my response was sharp.

"Let's do this, I have to pee."

"Oh my, did you tell the girls at the desk?"

"They knew."

"Honey, the restroom is right here. Go ahead!"

Now I was furious that they didn't tell me I could use the rest room. I assumed that I drank something for the test and they would need that in me for the test. I felt so much better afterwards and not as crabby. As we headed to the room that housed the CAT scan equipment, the tech who had to be in her late fifties asked about my cancer and listened while I gave her an abbreviated version of what happened. She asked if I had any metal on from the knee to waist, and I said just my jewelry. She made me remove my necklace but not the bracelets or earrings. She also asked if I had an underwire in my bra because if I did I would have to remove it. Then she asked if there were any metallic threads in my clothing or shoes. I had none of the above.

I saw her preparing an IV and thought I would speak up at that point about how sick I was from all medicines since the surgery and chemo.

"Everything makes me sick or I have a reaction with it." I figured I'd err on the side of caution here. I planned this on a Friday in case I was sick, so I would have two days to recover. She thought for a moment and put the contrast back in a cabinet and headed for another cabinet.

"I'm going to give you the dose I give to children. Hopefully, that will help. Also where was the bulk of your cancer located?"

"Most of it was in the pelvic region, obviously, but the little that remained after surgery was on the diaphragm."

"Well, the doctor only ordered a pelvic but I will shoot an extra one and try to cover that lower part of the diaphragm just to be safe."

I thought that she did a good job and was at least trying. I also couldn't figure out why the doctor didn't order a scan of the area right above the pelvic region. It made sense to me and the tech.

The tech then instructed me to lie on this table attached to a long large cylinder, all in white and about six-and-a-half feet tall and about five feet wide. It had a hole through its long center, and I saw tracks coming out and connected to the table I was about to lie on. She covered me with a blanket and asked me to shimmy my pants down to my knees so the zipper wouldn't show up. I remarked that the zipper was plastic but she said to just in case. I did as instructed and she came over to start the IV in my left arm.

"Butterfly needle."

"I can't do a butterfly on this. Hmm, this could be a problem." There was a long pause.

"I have one in the right arm that might work" I said trying to help. She untied the tourniquet and came around the table. I pointed to the one I thought would work.

"Yep, that will work." She carefully inserted the needle. *"Now you are going to smell alcohol and then taste metal. Tell me when both happen."* I told her when and told her that I was feeling sick.

"Stay with me Kim, and I'll get this done fast." She asked me to hold

the arm with IV up in the air (perpendicular to my body and to close my eyes and listen to the instructions. I closed my eyes as I heard her walk away and a door open and close. A moment later the table started to move, and the instructions started from an unknown female voice:

"Take a deep breath and hold it."

And then a few seconds later.

"Breath..."

I followed the instructions thankful I didn't have to hold my breath long.

The table moved back and forth a few times, and I could feel the outside of the CT machine as my raised arm would hit it every other move. After four times of holding my breath, I heard the tech say with a microphoned voice,

"You can put your arm down, Kim." I heard the door open and close again and footsteps coming towards me.

"I'm going to remove your IV now." I opened my eyes, and she was standing on my right side again. As she removed the IV, she told me I could redress. I did, and she walked me to the side counter where the girls were. I looked over at the waiting room through the glass and saw Chris sitting there.

"Your husband is waiting for you," one of the girls said and then right on top of that another one said,

"What kind of cancer do you have?"

I told her, and she asked a few more questions about the cancer. I answered all the questions and then took the opportunity to say, it's the chemo that causes nausea and not being able to eat for long periods of time makes it worse, that's why it's important to be on time with cancer patients.

"Oh, I didn't know that," the young girl said, and then a voice from behind me said:

"Also, if the patients are drinking contrast, they can use the rest room."

"Oh, I didn't know that either."

"Isn't that your job to know?" I couldn't help but blurt out. The tech immediately changed the subject to let me know that they would send the results to my doctor and to make sure I drank plenty of water for the rest of the day, and then she ushered me out.

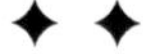

Four very long days later, I was sitting after work in my doctor's office. Once again, I waited and waited to be called back into a room. This time, I had Chris sitting next to me. I couldn't be upset about having to wait in this office, knowing that they had fit me in at the last minute, and I felt I would want that for anyone who was sitting where I was those many months ago. When they finally called me back, I went back alone, wanting to be able to ask the doctor questions and not have Chris almost pass out again.

When the doctor finally came through the doors, he held his arms open towards me. I got up from my chair in the corner and gave him a hug. He immediately sat down and opened the file. He re-read my diagnosis, and chemotherapy treatment to me, and I couldn't help but feel he was doing it more for his benefit than mine, to remind him who I was. He said that the CT scan showed no visible signs of cancer, and that I was effectively in remission, but that if my number goes up on the next CA125, he would have to hit me two more times with chemotherapy. He also told me that I had minor hydronephrosis. I asked what that was, and he drew a little picture showing me a kidney and a bladder with a tube that runs between them. He said that tube was hyper-extended or stretched out, and what he wanted me to do was see an urologist, and they would place a stent to fix it. I asked how something like that would happen, and the doctor was honest.

"I could have done it while I was checking everything for cancer."

I liked the fact that he didn't sweep it under the table or blame someone or something else. I had a list of questions of what I could and couldn't do. He told me: *"You should resume your normal life."*

Then, once again, like every other time, he took my hands in his and said it was and honor and a privilege. He walked out to the desk and said:

"Let's set her up with Dr. So-and-So and blood work monthly, and I'll see her here again in May."

I was standing behind him, and the one girl started typing into the computer. The doctor said goodbye again and headed to the next room. The girl behind the counter printed out a piece of paper with this new doctor's contact information. She handed it to me and sent me over to the girl who runs the office. She was already handing me a calendar and my script for the blood draws; one a month for the next three months.

"What if my number goes up?" I asked right away.

"Someone from the office will call you and have you come in to see the doctor."

Then I asked *"Can't you make me an appointment with this new doctor?"* Up until this point, she had made all my appointments, and this doctor was in the same building.

"No I can't for that particular doctor. You'll have to call."

I didn't want to call myself; I hated calling and making doctor's appointments. It irritated me…again. With a May return date, and no help with this new hydronephrosis I felt like I was being dismissed from their care with no life line.

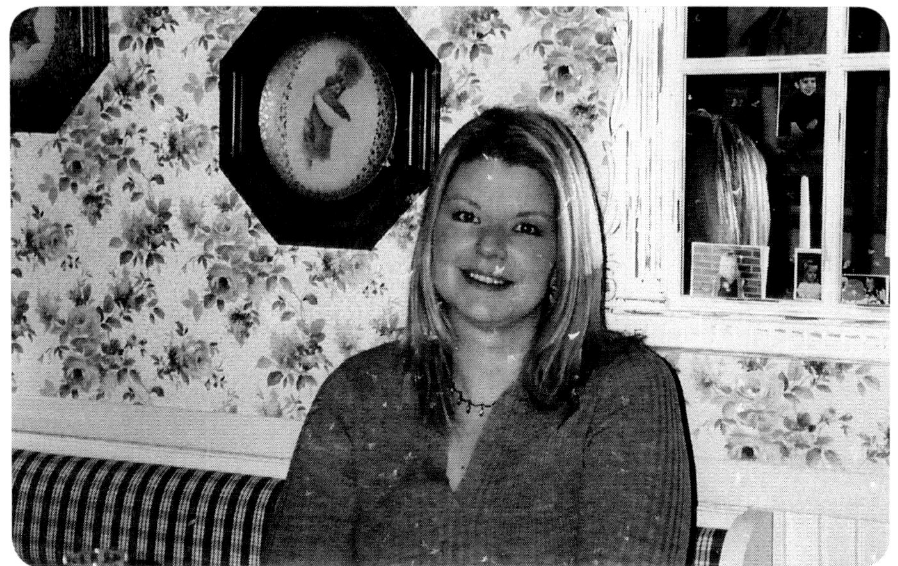

Me in 2003

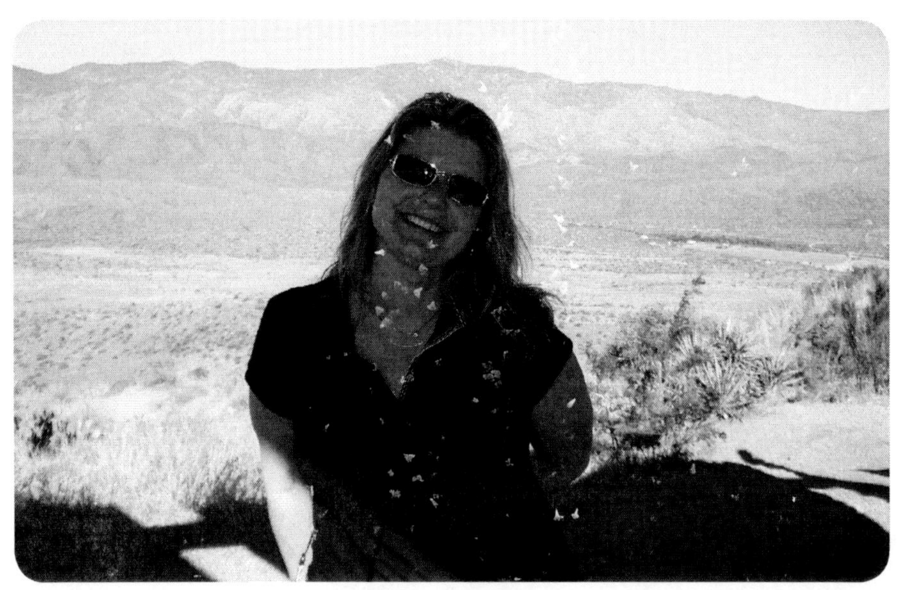

Me in 2006

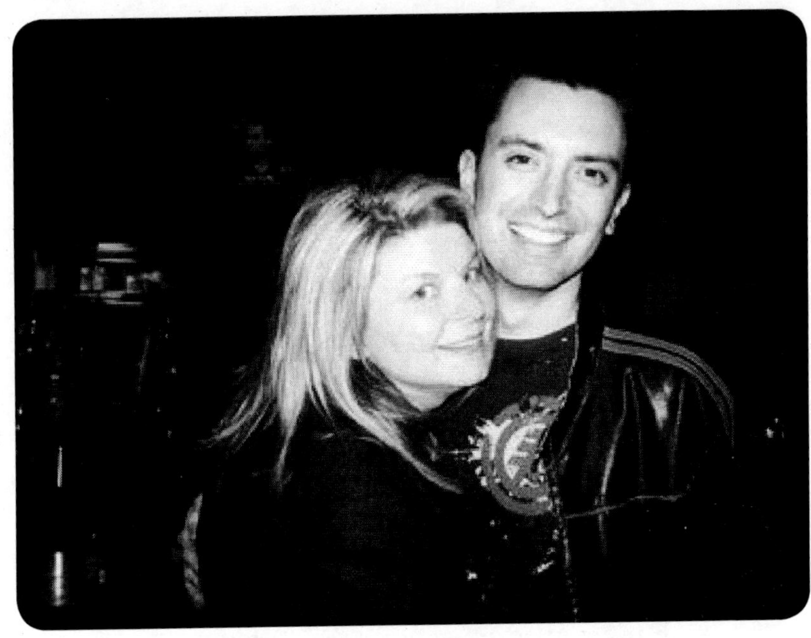

Chris and I 2008

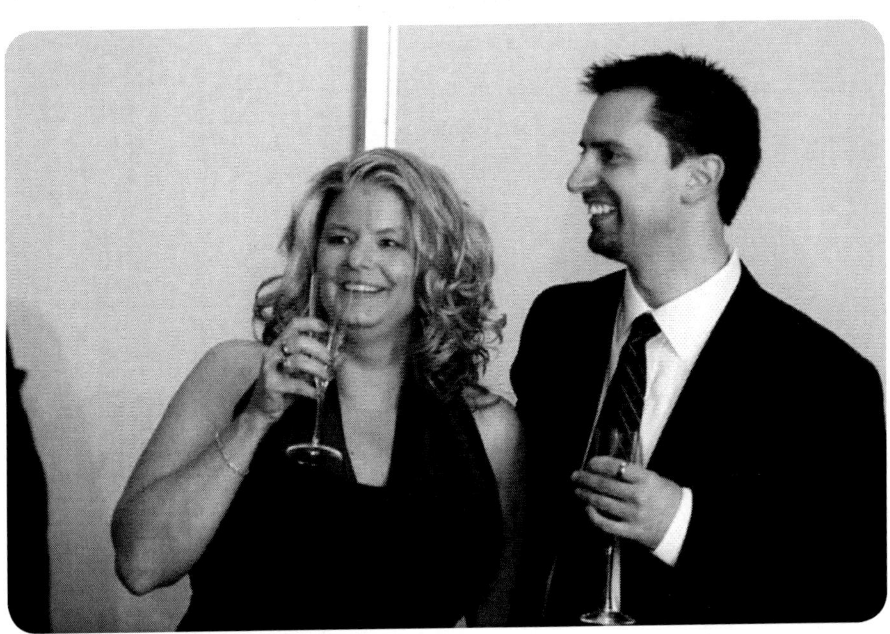

Chris and I at Charlotte and Sean's Wedding. September of 2009.

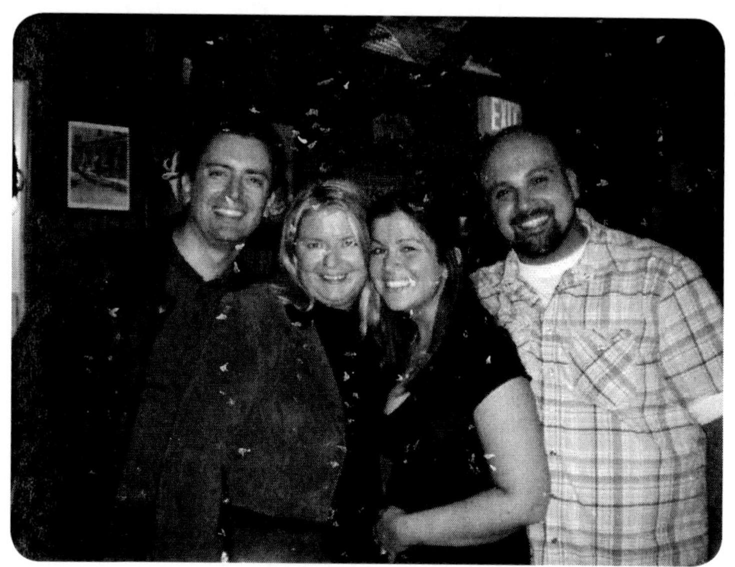

Chris and I with Jenn and Mike Balcom taken on the evening of their wedding. October 2009.

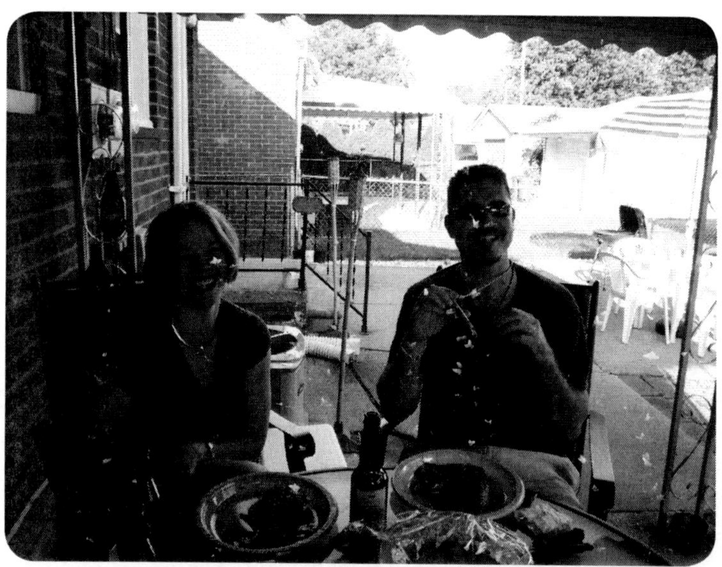

My BFF Charlotte Hobbs and my editor and Charlotte's husband Sean P. Hobbs.

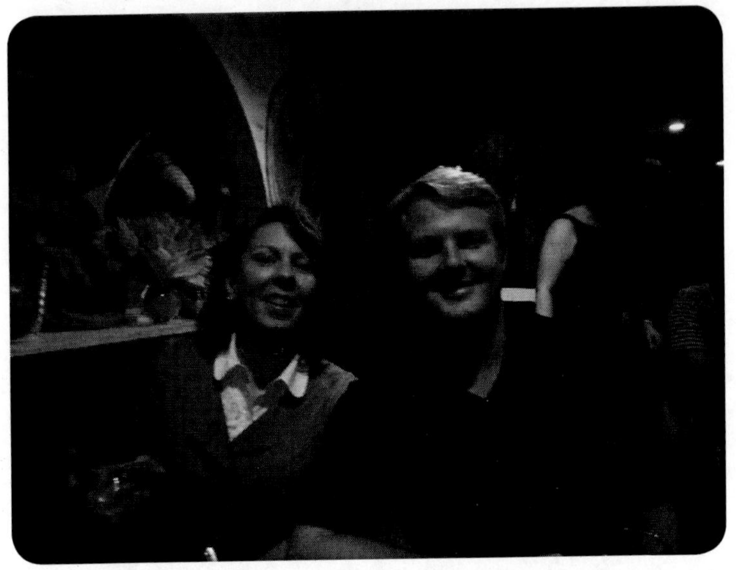

Danielle and Brian Webb. Our close friends and part of our large caregiver support system.

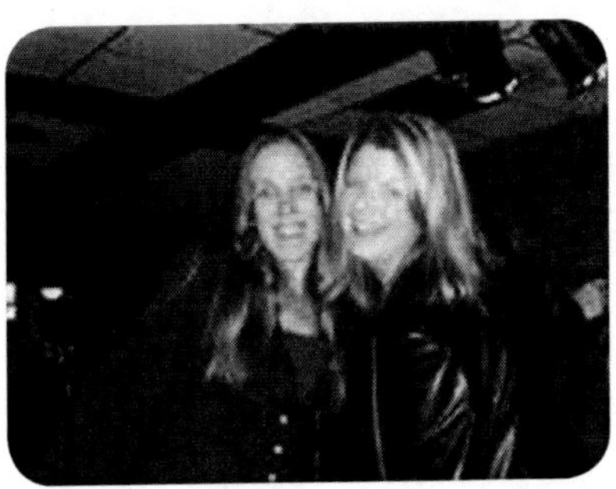

Me and Teri Selix (Teri is the founder of the "Think More Than Pink" nonprofit, supporting people with all kinds of cancer). This was taken at one of our many band events.

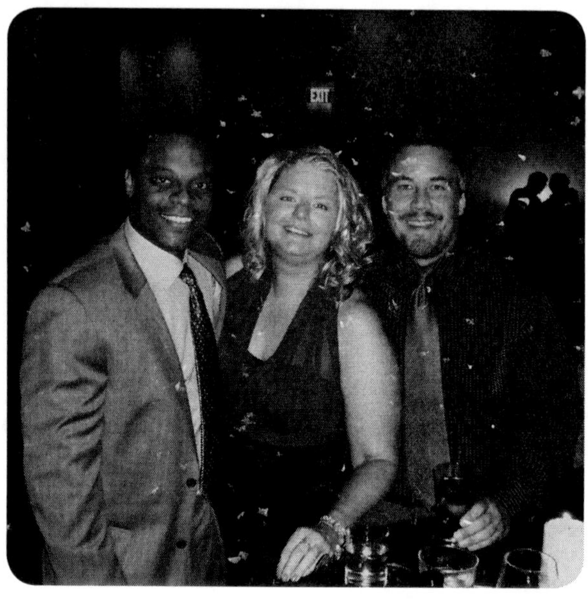

Me with my good friends David Chambers, and David Turski. I choose the picture because if you look closely at the midsection of my body you can see the 'weight gain' I thought I had. Just four months before this picture was taken, the dress I was wearing fit with room to spare. It is binding in this picture.

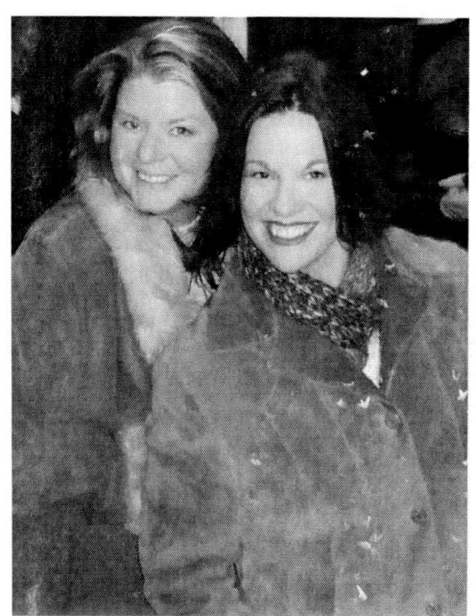

Me and Charlotte 2008

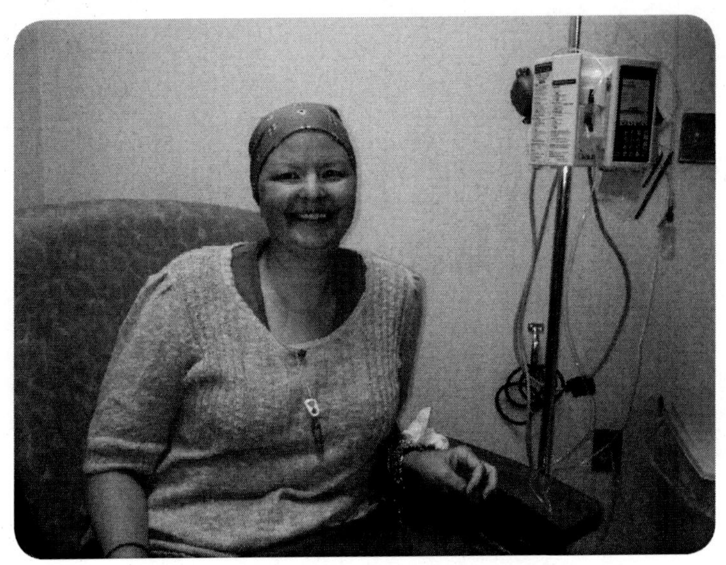

All Jacked in at the second cancer center

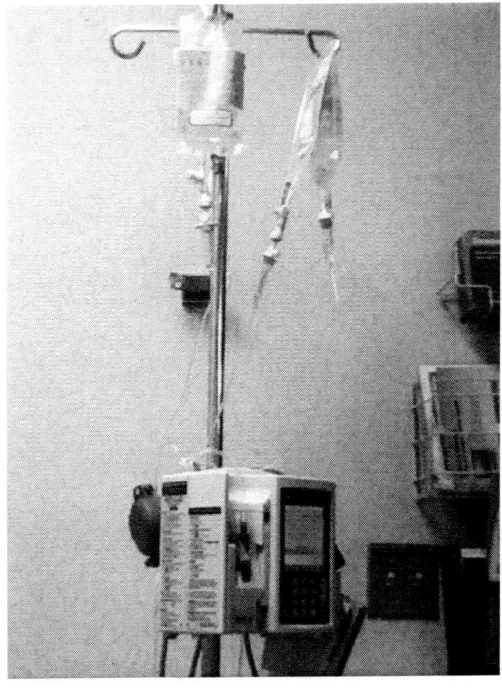

My IV pole

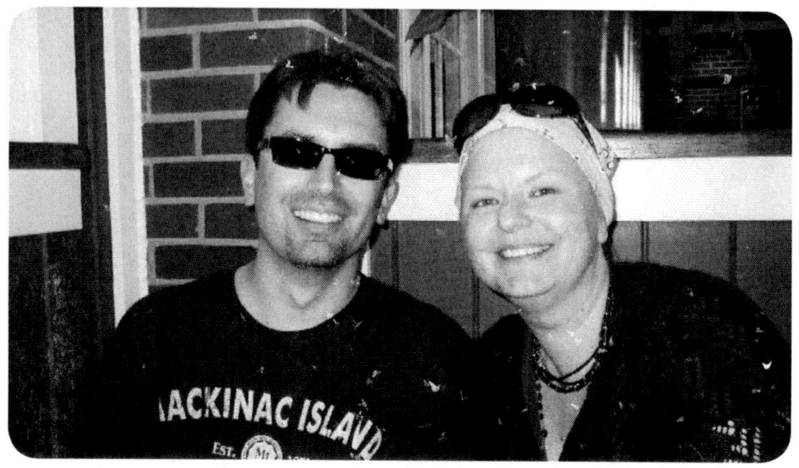

Me and Chris, one of the first times I let someone other than Chris photograph me without hair.

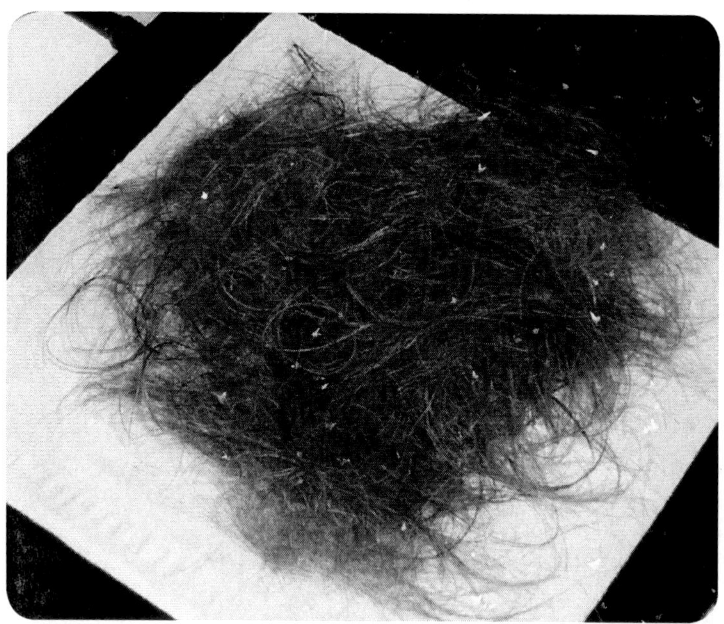

On the second round of chemo I wasn't afraid of my hair falling out. This was the first day it started to fall out (it was about 2 inches long) I kept combing it and piling it up.

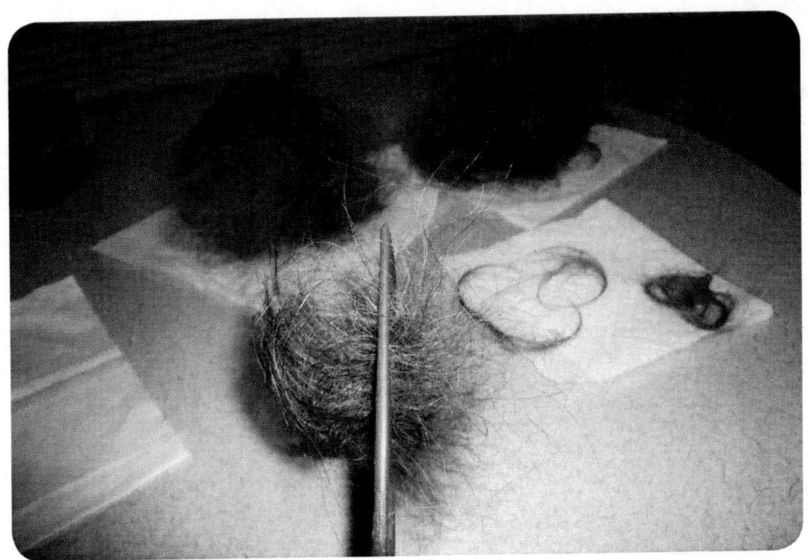

Very thin hair still falling out on the next day.

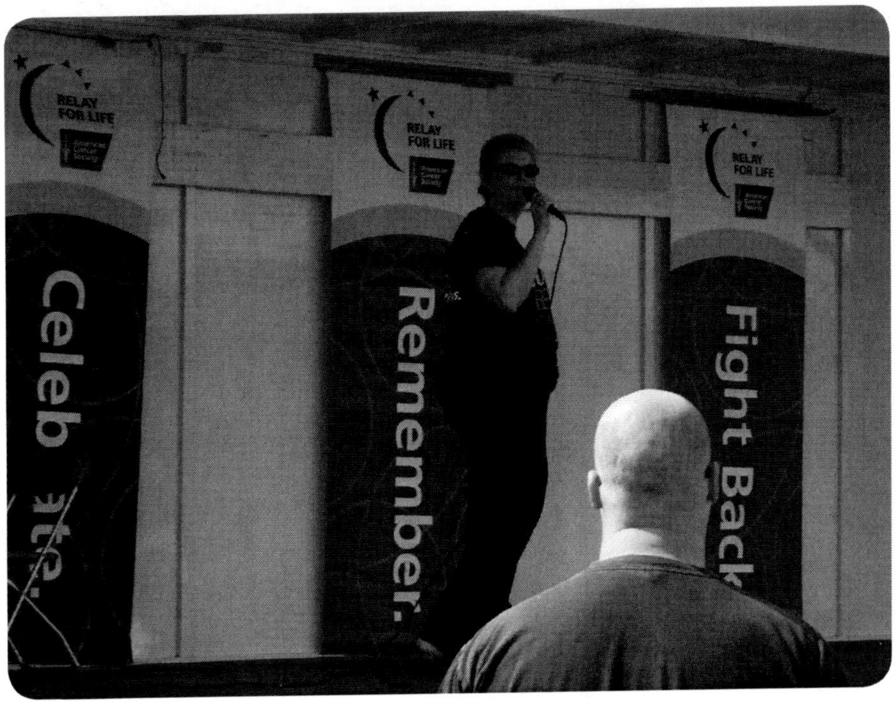

Giving my talk at the Taylor Relay for Life.

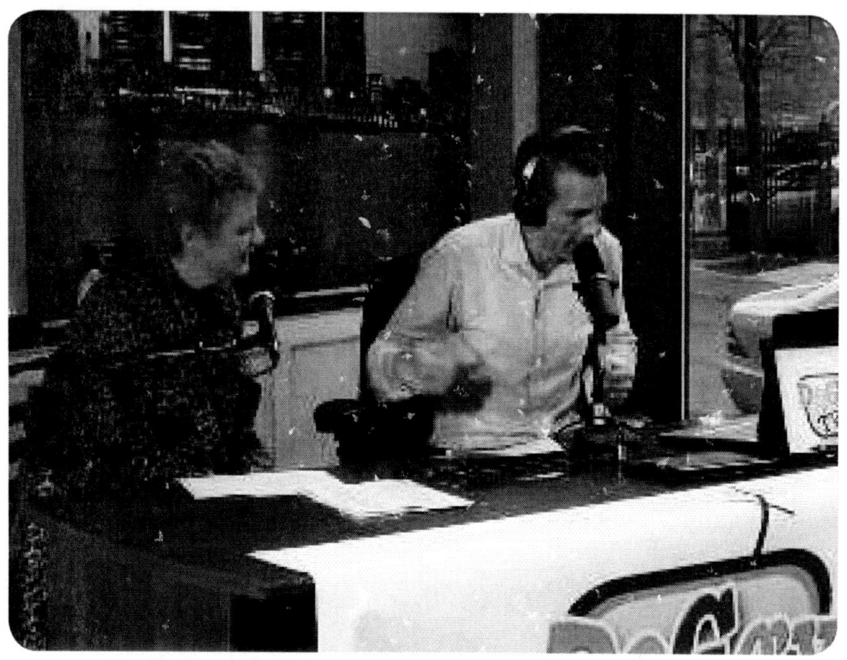

Radio interview before my Relay for Life speech with my brother-in-law Damon W. Perry.

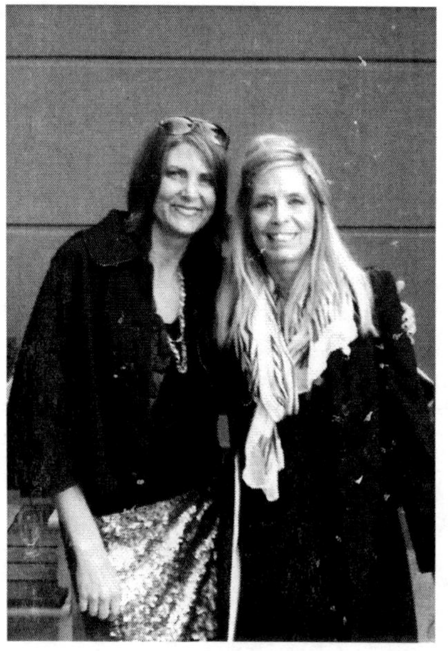

My sisters Jennifer Perry and Paula Lynch.

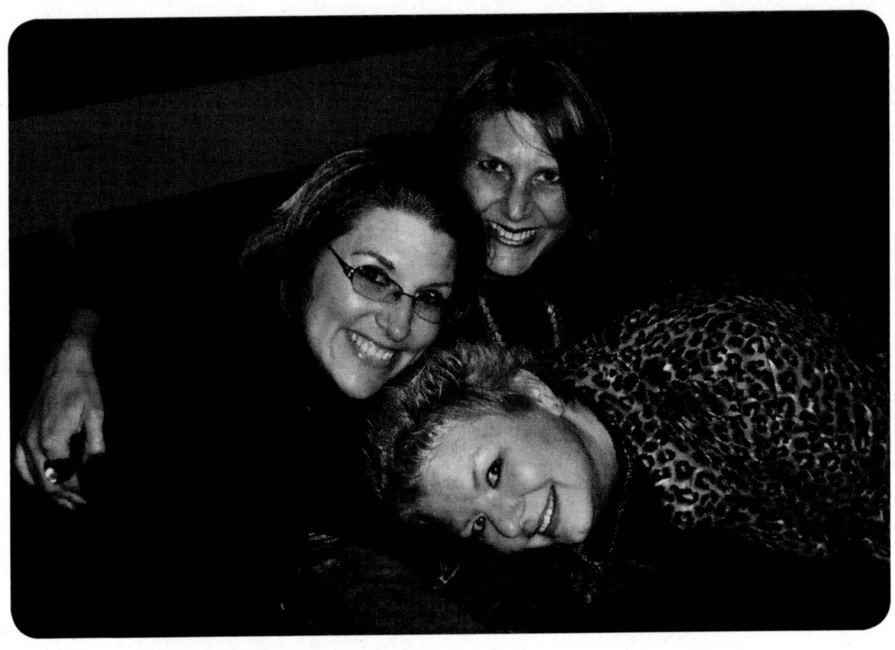

Me goofing off during remission with my sisters Michaelene Palyu and Jennifer Perry.

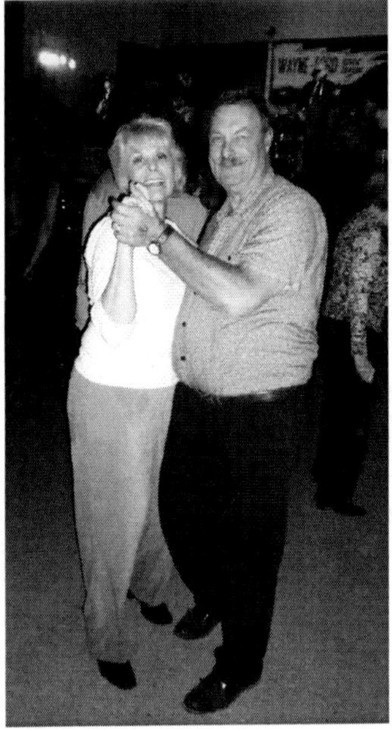

Chris's mom and dad.
Sue and Ken Vaughn.

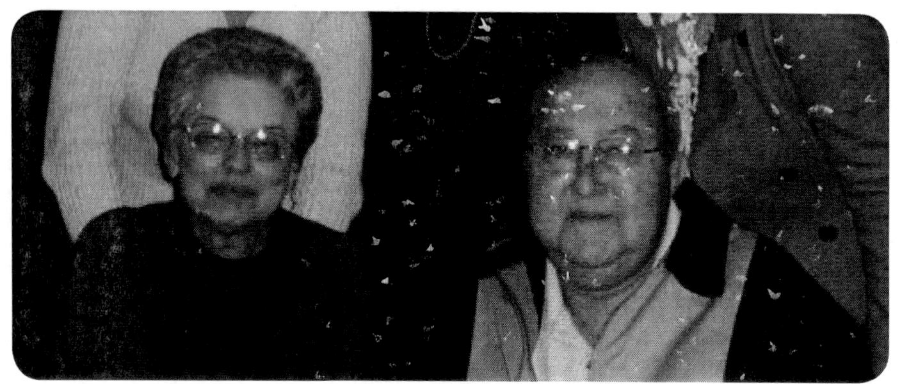

My parents Pat and Bob Allegrina (18 months into my dad's chemotherapy).

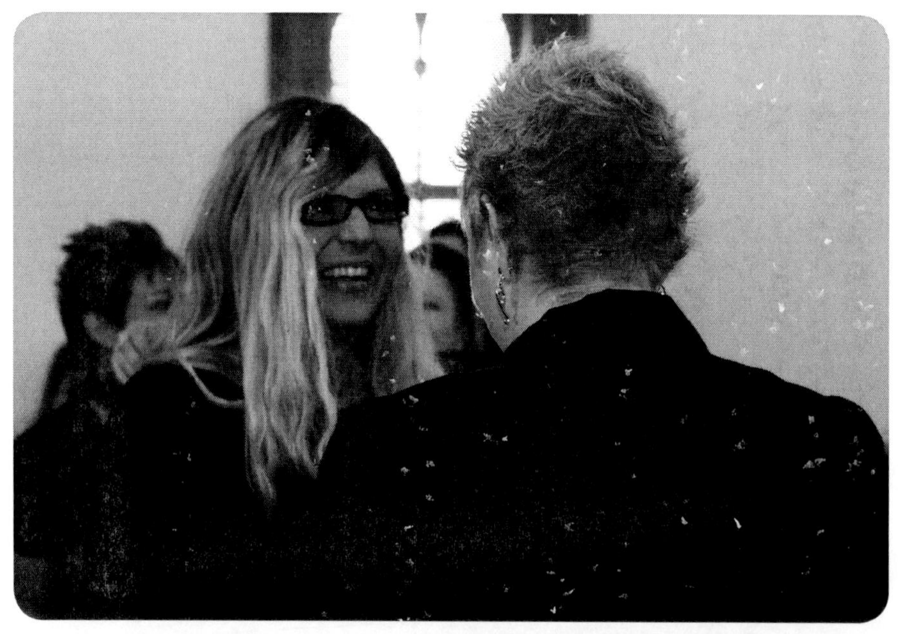

Andrea after radiation therapy. She always looked so fabulous! This was taken in April of 2011 at mine and Chris's wedding.

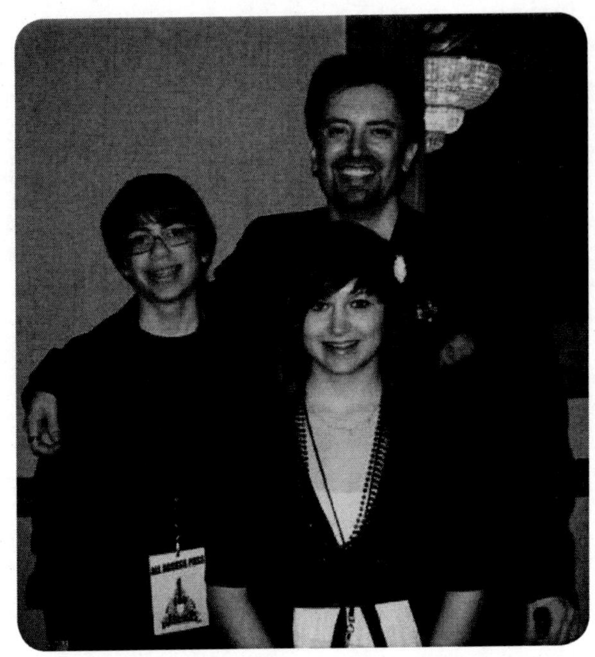

Chris, Kaitlin and Hunter (The Little Ones) on our Wedding day.

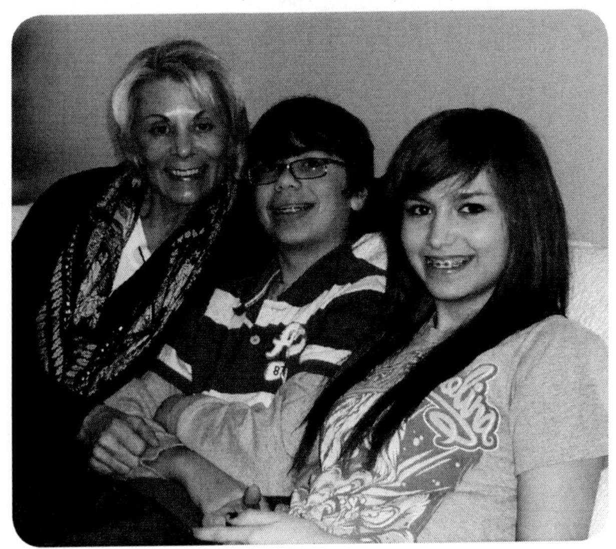

Sue with The Little Ones.

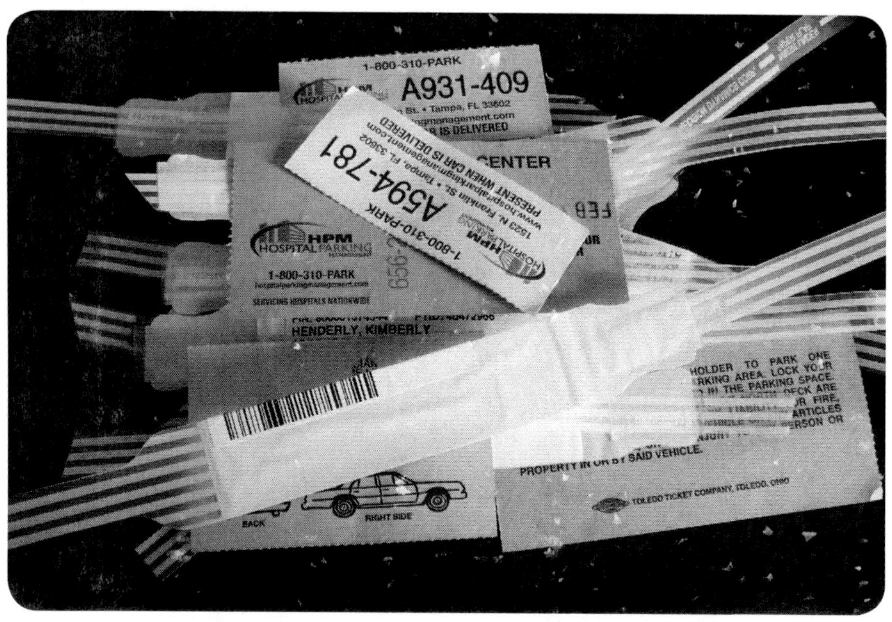

Some of the wristbands and parking passes from the multiple trips to the cancer centers.

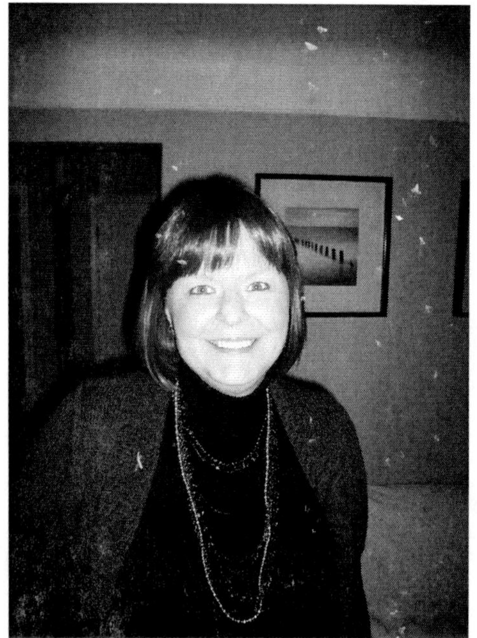

The Purple Wig is the favorite among my friends.

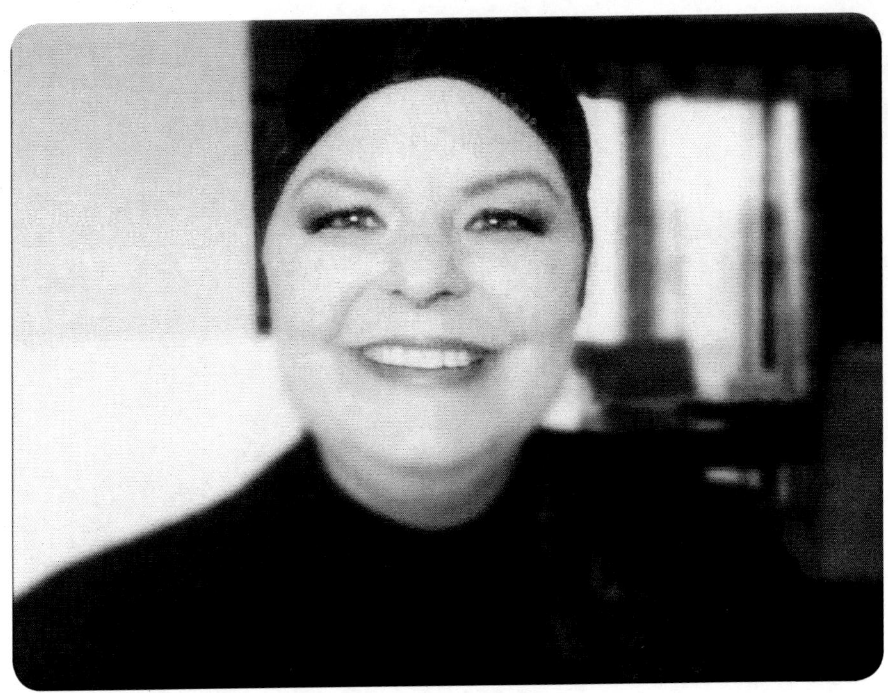

Had my friend Tina Craig a professional stylist and makeup artist do my makeup for a photo shoot. It was the only way I would agree to take off my headscarf and be photographed.

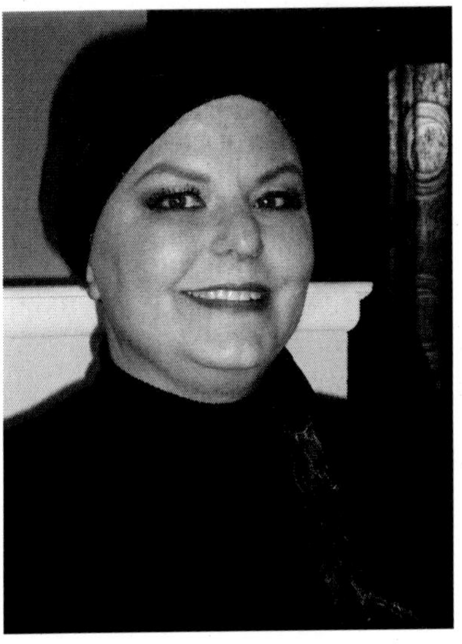

Same photo shoot.

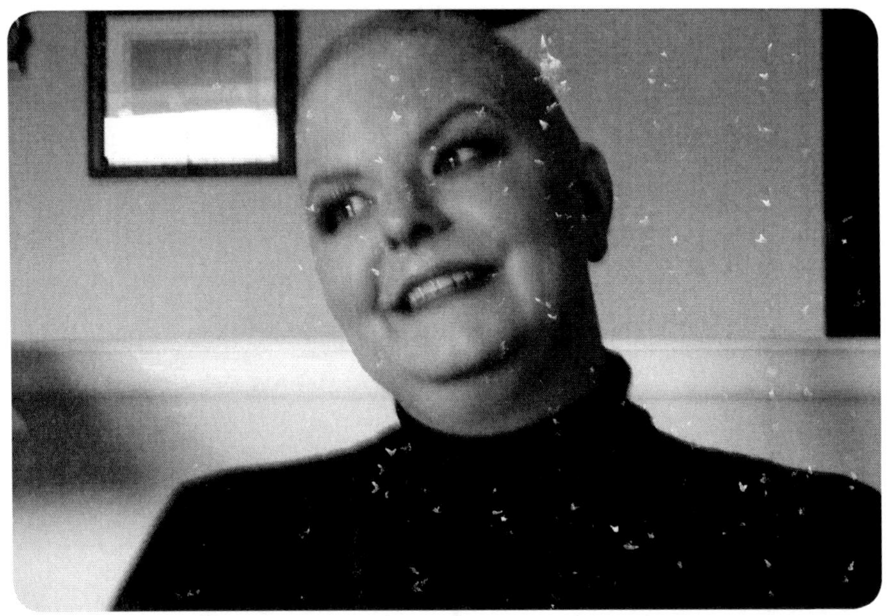

And here it is: one of the only photo's of me without a headscarf.

CHAPTER TWENTY-ONE
QUESTION EVERYTHING

The days started to pick up speed. Upon then news of remission, I immediately went to my social media page to let everyone know at the same time.

"REMISSION BITCHES" was all I had to put. As I reveled in all the congratulatory comments, offering to treat me to everything from-dinner, to drinks, with my favorite comment coming from the least expected person, always poised, highly intelligent, and spilling class from every cell, she is one of my most favorite people in the world, she commented back:

*"Write it down M***er f***ers."* I laughed so hard when I read that, and it felt good. Just to have it all behind me, to be able to move forward. I just had to get through the next couple months of blood draws to make sure the number stayed down, but I knew it would.

The next day at work, I was in the ladies' room after lunch to touch up my makeup, and I noticed my eyes for the first time in years I wasn't using Visine every day to get rid of the red. The whites of my eyes were white. I looked at my skin under the bright florescent bulbs, it was 'normal.' When I first started this job in April of 2009, I would come into this restroom and look in the mirror and keep trying to 'fix' my makeup, I thought I looked strange under the florescent lights. I blew it off at the time and blamed the lights, menopause, and the fact that my favorite makeup company discontinued producing makeup for the United States, and I couldn't order it from Europe. I thought I wasn't able to find the right powder. I bought all kinds of face lotions thinking that my skin was changing as I was aging. That red bloodshot eyes and shallow looking skin-tone with dark circles had been more signs that I had ignored and made up excuses for.

I looked at my skin, and I didn't really need a touch up, and those eyes—I felt like I did in my 20's… something I hadn't felt in a few years, I felt attractive. Even with the wig.

I was eating better. Oatmeal or egg whites for breakfast with an apple or an orange. For lunch on Sundays, I would cook five kinds of vegetables and then mix them together and take a container with the vegetables mixed with red wine vinegar, olive oil, pepper, garlic and turmeric. I had heard on Dr. Oz that this spice mixture of the pepper, garlic salt and turmeric was a cancer fighter and adding turmeric to cauliflower made it a super cancer fighter. I switched to drinking only brewed green tea with lemon and no more artificial sugar. I saved pop for special occasions, and I completely stopped drinking diet pop. This was huge for me as before the cancer diagnosis, I was consuming only diet pop and using artificial sweeteners. Every book on cancer I had read that was written by a cancer patient now in remission recommended taking all the chemicals out of your life. I ate a small amount of fish, chicken or turkey with dinner, and I still ate a lot of pasta and potatoes along with bread, substituting whole grains from the previous bleached flour. I couldn't seem to go without the carbs. I thought I was doing well—but I felt I could do better.

My vegetarian and vegan friends tried to coach me on things to eat, and the owner of my company who was on her own journey to find a healthy diet shared a tremendous amount of information and brought drinks and food in for me to try. She had a sweet tooth like myself and was always trying to find something for us to snack on in the afternoon when the cravings hit. I was willing to taste or try anything that I felt was 'good for me'. And it was nice to have someone around all day who understood that.

I knew it was time for the next step… the surgery had knocked me down to 201 at the lowest, but being on chemo and laying on the couch for six months had sent my weight right back to 222. I was down twenty some pounds. I assumed most of it was the masses they removed, but I knew I needed to get some of this weight off. I looked on the hospital website and found three nutritionists associated with the hospital. On my lunch hour, I walked down to the café in our building and called the first one. After speaking to her on the phone and telling her my story and what I wanted to do, she actually suggested that I call the person who was second on my list to call saying she worked closely with cancer patients. I called her and repeated the same story. She agreed to see me and said she could help; I made an appointment for after work a few days later and she said she was going to send me a questionnaire to fill out. The three page form was in my inbox when I got back to my desk.

While I was in the café that day eating lunch and making phone calls, I also called the urologist's office. This was my second call to the office; the first one I had made the day after my doctor's visit on the way home from work. The office was closed and the message relayed the office hours. I was calling during the specified hours and this time I got an 'out to lunch' recording and instructions to call back. This is why I hated making doctor's appointments!

A week later, I would call again this time on a Friday and for some reason they were closed on that day also, even though the recording actually said they were open. I gave up, went online, and found another urologist, called and told them what the issue was, they said someone would call me back. The girl on the phone did ask if I had any type of infection, bladder, urinary tract, or kidney. I said I didn't and she suggested I go as long as I could without the stent because once I got it, it would be a life-time issue and there was pain involved with a stent. I didn't have to go in, and I didn't have to have another procedure according to this person, so I was good.

After I hung up I didn't think about it again and nobody called me back from the office. It had only been six weeks and the laziness when it came to doctor's was already setting in. After having the hysterectomy and going through chemo, my peeing habits didn't really change. I was still going to the bathroom several times a day. I made no real effort to question or follow-up further with anyone at either urologist office.

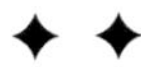

I met with my nutritionist. She read over my question and answer sheet and didn't really have much to say. I told her about all my failed weight loss attempts of the past and what I had changed my diet to.

She suggested a diet supplement drink they sold in the pharmacy at the hospital. I looked at the bag she showed me and the first thing I noticed was all the chemicals in the ingredient list. Then, I noticed soy was also on the list. Can I have soy having had a gynecological cancer? She didn't know.

I was thinking I would get someone I could come and see once a week and go over my diet and they would make suggestions and coach me through. After telling this person my thoughts, she suggested a different program. It was meant for people who were going to go through bariatric surgery. She gave me a contact number. Again, no answers and no help from this hospital. Yet because this nutritionist was connected to the cancer center, she was able to charge a pretty penny to my insurance company, and I had no new information to help me with nutrition and weight loss. I was maintaining my 222 lb. weight, but even with all the vegetables, it wasn't dropping. Where were all the groups I read about in these books? Where was all the assistance, the advice, the help. I felt like I was floundering all alone. I knew what I was experiencing at this hospital/cancer center wasn't living up to the hype. I was starting to get frustrated.

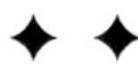

As I moved through the month of February, I started to notice more and more changes with my body. I was starting to build my energy back up. My bathroom issues had all disappeared, and I was getting back to normal being able to poop every morning again. My eyelashes, eyebrows and hair started to grow back slowly. My eyebrows came back the fastest. After eight weeks from the last chemo treatment, they were almost completely back to their original shape. I was happiest to see my eyelashes slowly come back, and when they were all in, I realized how much they had thinned in the two years leading up to my diagnosis. I thought the loss of some eyelashes was normal as I aged; again another missed sign. It took a full three months before I would go out without some type of covering on my head. The first time I did, my hair couldn't have been longer than a half-inch. I added some gel and tried to style it. I wasn't good with short hair, so

I Google-imaged very short hair and thousands of pictures came up. I did the best I could that weekend in March and headed to lunch with Chris and to walk around the mall to get some much needed exercise. I was starting to feel so much better. I was incredibly happy that day as we talked about rescheduling the wedding. We made plans over lunch and picked a date, April 30th. With only about seven weeks to go, I went into over-drive planning the wedding at a local chapel with a cocktail party immediately following. We wanted that same fun Vegas experience and with my background in hospitality I knew I could pull it off.

I yanked my dress out of the bag and tried it on. It barely fit and the shop had totally screwed up the added-on straps, but it was 'good enough.' That whole it-has-to-be-perfect-gene within me was gone. I told my three close friends what we were doing and to add whatever they wanted to the red sundresses they had bought for Vegas to make it warmer for an April wedding in Michigan, and we'd be good. The Tommy Bahama style shirt the guys were going to wear with shorts in the ninety degree dessert heat was also replaced with a black suit and whatever they wanted to wear for shirt and shoes. We dubbed it "The Rock n Roll Wedding" with Chris being Mr. Rock and me being Mrs. Roll. Once again, I let myself get incredibly excited about the whole thing. I felt the old Kim coming back—I had to watch my every move from what I did in the way of exercise and work to what went in my mouth.

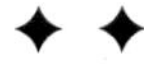

Heading into April, I started to notice things; this time being so aware of all the 'signs' that were laid before me and that I ignored, I tried not to ignore them this time. The swollen glands, the gastric intestinal issues, and then came the inability to swallow food correctly: it would lie in a lump in what seemed like a position right at the top of my lungs. Then, the tiredness started. Hardly noticeable at first, just a feeling like you wanted to doze off at your desk. Not being able to get through the entire day, like maybe you had a little bug or something. When they started to creep back in ninety days after my final chemo, in the back of my head, I knew what was coming on the next blood test. I had it all figured out in my head… the first month was recovery from the final chemo; the second month had me bouncing around like a kid trying to do anything and everything I could. I pushed with that thought into March. Even went ahead and set the date for my wedding and made plans. I was in those first months living on what the doctor had said *an 80/20 chance of chemotherapy working*. In my mind, it meant I was completely done, never having to deal with it again. I knew however, that these symptoms were all present pre-surgery and not present after surgery until April of 2011. I went to not one but three tarot readers, all who said by June I would be fine. I kept a happy, positive tone with everyone. I'm doing better, good and bad days, I would say. Then, in about mid-April, I was sitting on the couch eating and the pasta and vegetable dish I had made myself for dinner got stuck in my digestive tract. This hadn't happened since the months leading into the diagnosis. I went to the bathroom in that familiar pattern and coughed it out. *Don't panic,* I said to myself, *it's a little dry; you aren't drinking pop to wash stuff down anymore.* Then, it happened a second and third time in April. I went back to very small bites followed by lots of water, so everything would wash down. The intestinal distress came next; I found myself hiding Tums in my lunch box again, taking two at a time to try and stop it. The CA125 in February and March were twenty-four and then sixteen. I took my next CA125 on April 12th at the port flush the next day. I asked the nurse doing the port flush to check my number so I wouldn't have to call the doctor's office. It had jumped from sixteen back up to twenty-five. I knew I was doomed at that moment, I made my next port flush appointment and left. I burst into tears in my car and drove back to work; ready to pretend nothing had happened. I called The Other from the parking lot, in his usual boost-me-up, don't-worry-fashion, he calmed me down, so I could work. At that moment, I decided to tell no one else about the jump.

It was about two weeks later when both the glands in my neck started to swell. It had happened numerous times leading up to the cancer diagnosis. The two most notable sent me to the doctor. But this was an underlying, never quite normal kind of swelling; it was just there, in my neck, on both sides. So, I sat, four months out of chemo, and symptoms were recurring, but I had a bigger problem this time... Could I take the chemo again? The monthly battle of the pain. Vomiting uncontrollably and then shitting myself was so incredibly fresh in my mind... The doctor said in February, he would hit me twice more if the numbers went up. I knew I could. It would suck, but at least I know what to do now. I also knew I could time this, so I could take vacation days. There's the crux of the matter—my job. Things were just getting back to normal for me at work. I loved what I was doing, and looked forward to moving ahead with the company. How was I going to prove I was a team player and in it for the long haul if I had to go back again for chemo? I thought about all the people who kept their cancer a secret from everyone. I knew the owner was sympathetic, but there was still a business to run. Hence, the decision to keep it to myself for these two rounds I was sure I was going to have to endure.

Our wedding on April 30th went off without a hitch. The Rock and Roll wedding of the year!

Months later, people were still talking about it. I was on a high from all the activity and excitement. Summer was fast approaching in Michigan, and for those who are lifers here, the season is short. If you are really lucky, you can squeak in good weather from mid-May to the end of September. I had missed the lion's share of the summer of 2010, and I was ready for summer.

The Other and I started to make our weekly plans. The weekends filled up fast: going to see friends and family, trying to get my wind back for working out. I had almost forgotten about all the signs that were creeping up on me.

I started drinking coffee and Mountain Dew again to keep up with all that I wanted to do. At the beginning of May, I had another scheduled doctor's appointment. I went alone and was ready with the questions. I told him what the urologist office I had talked to said, and he agreed. It could wait until there was an infection to contend with.

Then I told him about the symptoms and the jump of the CA125 from the teens into the twenties. His answer:

"Don't worry. It's under thirty-five. I could take samples on the same day from both arms and get two different numbers. We go by those numbers."

I talked myself into being relieved at that statement. However, something nagged at me over that increase.

I went to leave and the girl behind the desk handed me my script for my next blood draw and doctor's appointment along with a CT scan. They were all scheduled for the end of August. I questioned not getting the CA125 monthly. I really wanted to make sure that the number did not go up again. Twenty-six is not far from thirty-five.

"It's protocol. Six months in a row then every three months for a couple of times then every six months. Soon it will be only once a year!" She answered the question and looked at the resident doctor standing at the other end of the desk. *"Correct?"* She was looking for backup in her comment.

"Yes. That's the way everyone does it."

"What if I wanted blood drawn monthly just to be on the safe side?" I remarked.

"It's not necessary," the resident said in a dismissive tone.

These were the people I had chosen to handle my life at this point, and my faith in them was slowly slipping away. I loved the attitude of my doctor. He was so upbeat, and I *thought* direct about what he thought, and as The Other pointed out over and over, he had saved my life. I had to trust him and his staff. I felt like I had nowhere else to go, and I was really at a loss of what should be done and what needed to be done. More internet research? Talking to friends with cancer? I felt like I had tapped all those resources.

I left the office that day happy that I didn't have to return for three months. Even though there was this underlying feeling that I should be questioning these people more, I pushed that feeling away and went about my life.

CHAPTER TWENTY-TWO
A CANCER VETERAN

It was May of 2011, when Teri Selix, my friend and fellow cancer veteran, had contacted me back in February at the start of my official remission. Teri was heavily involved in the Taylor, MI Relay For Life. The Taylor Relay was one of the largest in the State, and it was her calling when it came to her own cancer survival. "Think More Than Pink" is her slogan and nonprofit organization. Her Team, "Rocker Chicks," recently changed to "The Rockers," reflected her love of music and her involvement in band promotion. I had met Teri through my band management. She used to come to the shows and eventually was recruited to do a promotional packed for one of my bands. Our friendship grew, and when I was diagnosed, she was always a text or email away with answers to questions that I had at all times of the day and night. She had tried to recruit me to be part of the Relay Team explaining that the money raised was for The American Cancer Society and supported all cancers, not just breast cancer. In my internet surfing over the last several months, I had come to realize that the biggest money-making machines were strong-arming many well-meaning people. I wasn't happy with the whole fundraising thing, and even the cancer center I had first contacted when this whole mess started, the one who told me "we're not a question and answer line," had sent me fundraising materials! I didn't like any of it especially since *not one organization stepped up to help me with anything*! I had to depend on family and friends.

Teri had a different idea. Having heard me speak at my party in November, she asked if I would be interested in giving "The Survivor's Speech" at the opening ceremonies. I was shocked and thrilled. I had been talking over the last couple of months to friends and family about needing to get the word out on chemotherapy and how bad it was. This was a selfish chance to make some connections, and start spreading the word. I knew I was a good public speaker having won oratorical contests in high school. I've spoken at my sisters' and friends' weddings and other events. I knew I could make an impact. I agreed, and she gave me the contact information for the woman in charge of setting up that part of the ceremonies.

We worked out the details and she gave me a five minute timeline to tell 'my story.' I knew that in five, short, minutes, I had to get out not just my story but remind all the survivors how much we all had suffered and get the point across that this was all completely unacceptable. It only took me forty minutes to write the speech, and I had been practicing it in Chris' studio using his microphones and PA system to get used to addressing people in that matter. The date was approaching, and that May morning was sunny and beautiful. Chris, Hunter and I arrived early and we couldn't believe the set up.

The band Chris and I had been involved with in the years leading up to my diagnosis had played a Relay for Life once.

Back then, we were on a stage facing a high school track and there were a dozen tents set up in the middle of the track with a couple dozen people walking around. We played several songs, and people liked the music, but it didn't seem like that big a deal to me and I used to think that all of these Relays should be combined to make it more fun with more people participating.

When we pulled up to the set area in the park for this Taylor Relay For Life, I was amazed. A small tent city had already been erected. There were dozens and dozens of tents, and each one had a stand set up selling some type of craft or service to raise not just the money from walking but additional money. The set up was twenty times the size of the Relay the band had played for. I checked in at the first tent I saw. It had tables and chairs in place for a luncheon, and I found the woman I was supposed to talk to. She gave me a special shirt to wear and Chris and Hunter caregiver pins. We exchanged our stories, and she told me where the bandstand was and when to meet her there. At the end of my speech, I would walk around the path one time leading the Relayer's for the start of the walk. I headed off to look around and found Teri's tent set up in a shaded corner of the track. She gave me details and Chris helped her do a little set up. I thought that next year, my blog could sponsor her with money and signs because by next year, I would have been back at work for a full year, and we would have extra to spend and donate to her team.

We headed out to see the other tent set ups. Such creative people with great ideas to raise money. It was very carnival-like and upbeat. I was starting to realize there were hundreds and hundreds of people here. My sister Jennifer came with my little nephews Nathan and Gavin to watch and so did Charlotte and Sean, with their small son Colin, and I was so happy when I saw Sean's mom who was in from California had also decided to come. Chris's band mate and BFF and his wife and their new baby Ben were also in attendance. I smiled at Mike; he was our lead singer and had been the lead singer in another band I had managed previously. He looked at me and gave me great advice on how to command the stage when I spoke. I smiled knowing he had played out last night and was probably only running on a couple hours of sleep; when I mentioned that, he said, *"only for you Kim."* I was so happy to see his wife Jenn. We had been IM-ing, emailing and texting for months. She had a very rough last couple of months of her pregnancy and was couch-bound when I was couch-bound with chemo. I felt like I had someone who understood the despair of sitting there day after day not being able to move because they were too sick. Now, we finally had a chance to see each other face to face and hug. Brian showed up, with his daughter Brooke who was always a ray of sunshine for me. As she ran up, she yelled, *"MISS KIM! MISS KIM!"* and hugged me.

The local high school band was playing on one side of stage and people were gathering. All the chairs were full and people were standing to the back and on the sides of the stage. I had never spoken in front of this many people, but I felt confident going into this speech with all my friends there. They gave me strength. I thought I would be speaking to them, something I did all the time, and it made me comfortable. Chris set up the video camera because I wanted to see how I looked speaking and mostly because I wanted to hear what I wrote. I kissed and hugged Chris and turned to head towards the back of the stage.

Hunter looked at me and said, "*You got this.*" I knew I would do great at that moment.

I listened as the head of the Relay Organization from our area spoke, along with the mayor of Taylor. They gave props to all the sponsors, and then the lady I had been dealing with came on the stage to introduce me. I insisted she make mention that I like to call myself a Cancer Veteran. I didn't like the word Survivor. Although good for some, I felt like we were in a war with this crazy disease. I walked out praying I wouldn't trip. Just like I had rehearsed in the basement, I used the move I had stolen from the majority of stand-up comics I had seen. I grabbed the microphone and set the stand behind me in one smooth move. It was my time ...... Here's what I said...

Like Barb said, my name is Kim Henderly and I am a Cancer Veteran. I like to call myself a veteran because a tiny little cell in my body amassed troops and staged a mutiny if you will, so I flipped them off, told them to bite me ***and they did*** *and I waged war.*

Now this all started a few years ago when I noticed some things going on...

My hair was thinning
Had a little weight gain around the middle
Night sweats
and I was feeling tired

So I went to ***not one*** *but* ***two doctors****, who both looked me in the eye and said*

You're menopausal.... so I feel this way 'cause I'm OLD?

But Doc listen-I used to be able to get up at five,
Work out for an hour,
Go to work for nine hours,
Come home, take care of the house,
Make dinner,
Do some gardening,
Go on the computer,

Watch TV,

Go to bed at midnight and get up the next day at 5am and start the process over....

Now I'm sleeping ten hours a day and mainlining caffeine!!

Well... you know... you are not twenty anymore!

Not 20! I don't want to be twenty, I was a moron in my twenties, but I would like to feel like I did at forty-five?

They both dismissed me.

It wasn't long after that that I was sitting on the couch doing nothing. I went to get up and I couldn't move 'cause the pain in my lower left side was paralyzing. And just to let you know my pain tolerance, I had dry socket with a wisdom tooth and didn't take any additional pain killers or have it repacked. In our house we call that 'cowboy up,' work through the pain. And, because I have a propensity to do stupid things like that, my Other enlisted the help of his mom to make sure I got to the doctor's the next day. On the ride over, she asked me what I thought I had....

"Gosh, I hope it's not kidney stones!"

Who would have thought that was the lesser of the two evils?

So I got a cute young nurse practitioner who did a thorough exam and announced happily that I was twenty-two weeks pregnant!

How can that be? I'm menopausal!

But she insisted, and I insisted that I was forty-seven and knew how to not *get pregnant. So for the first time in my life, a CA125 and a trans-vaginal ultra-sound were ordered. The CA125 numbers were through the roof and the ultrasound showed a twenty-two centimeter mass... then she told me to see a general surgeon and kicked me out of the office without being able to talk to a doctor... Ever try to find a doctor on Fourth of July weekend? Well that was the task put to my mother-in-law, and she found me a doctor...*

I'd like to say this about my doctor... ever been watching TV and said, "Why can't I find a doctor like that?" That's my doctor! So he looked at all my tests and seven days later he was wheeling me in for major surgery. I woke up from that surgery five hours later, eight body parts short and a diagnosis of ovarian cancer. That's right I drew the short straw. Not only did I have one of the deadliest cancers around, I was already stage III. *So before I could heal from surgery, they installed a port and started me on chemotherapy.*

Now chemo there's a treat huh! Laying on the bathroom floor trying to figure out which foods will actually stay inside your body. Legs twitchin' all over the place in pain. Hands and feet going numb. Sucking on ice to keep the mouth sores down. All while you get the watch your hair go down the drain. Yeah, we wouldn't treat prisoners like this. Yet it seems to be ok to treat a cancer patient this way.

There is a long black granite wall in Washington DC called the Vietnam Memorial Veterans Wall; and not to take away from those who gave their lives in service of this country, but that wall is five hundred feet long...

About a football field and a half. Got a mental picture?

It would take ten *of those walls* once a year *to list the names of all the people who died fighting our war...*

Lewis Black said it best... (I pulled my phone out of my pocket imitating him)

This is not just a phone: it's a computer, no wires.

The greatest minds in the world have spent the last thirty years working on this *(I held out my phone)*

Now I don't care how big your support group is, and mine is huge. These people have helped me financially, emotionally, and physically, but what we need is these great minds working on our war*!*

And that takes money! That's why we're all here today!

Give generously folks.

If you've enjoyed these caffeine induced ramblings you can catch more of them at kimhenderly.com... my name is Kim Henderly, and I am a 142 day cancer veteran!

With that final statement, I turned to hand the microphone to the lady that introduced me, and I heard the applause. I could pick out the yelling and cheering from my friends in the crowd. I prayed that they got it. That the humor I had tried to interject had made it easier to hear. I wanted to cry, but as I left the back of the stage I was grabbed by Teri to hold a sign and start the walk. As I heard the lady announcing the start of the relay with the survivors walk and as people fell into line behind us, I noticed Suzi being pushed in a wheelchair next to us. She was happy, and told me she loved my speech. Suzi is related to Teri. Cancer and its treatment had done a number on her and so many members of her family. She was so happy that day. I didn't know it at the time, but even though we would email for the next few months and comment on each other's social networks, in just nine short months she would fall victim. Another warrior in the war on cancer lost.

CHAPTER TWENTY-THREE
LONDON BRIDGE IS FALLING DOWN, FALLING DOWN

The summer progressed without incident; I made Chris put my speech on-line and showed it to everyone I could, trying to get my message out. My hair grew enough for me to head to the salon for some color. People had told me that my hair would be different. It was. It reminded me of being in my teens, thick and healthy, like it used to be before years of changing the color and the perms of the 80's; the left front quarter was growing in a weird bent fashion. I assumed it was because the chemicals destroyed the cells, and they were growing back a bit damaged. As my nails grew out, you could see the wave or ridges that had formed while on chemotherapy, and the new smooth nail that was coming in behind it. Against my better judgment, I caved and started getting manicures and then shellac manicures. Poisons and chemicals being absorbed into my scalp from hair-color, and nails and the surrounding area with the manicure polish and nail polish remover. I was getting sloppy about paying attention to things like that. I tried to remember to wear a mask when cleaning the house and using chemicals or working in the garden, but I soon got lazy about all that also.

Then it happened. I was showering. It was mid-July and I felt a lump between my legs. I started to cry. We had promised The Little Ones a summer weekend with us, and I wanted to honor that. So I said nothing and went on with our weekend. On Sunday morning, I was like a caged animal pacing and waiting for Chris to drive The Little Ones back to their mom's homes. He usually was early about arriving anywhere but today he was enjoying his morning and in no hurry. As soon as he got in the car with the kids, I closed the windows and blinds in our room and screamed and cried until I heard his car pull back in the drive.

He came in the house calling my name and walked around the corner from the living room and saw me on the bed. He sat down and asked what was wrong. I told him about the lump I found and we sat on the bed and hugged and cried together. It felt good to lie on the bed in his arms. I wanted the moment to go on forever. It felt better in that spot—like nothing could touch me. We spent the rest of the day alone, talking, trying to plan our next step which I knew was a lost cause. There was obviously no future planning when you have cancer. That night I took the script out of my wallet for the CA125 and changed the date to upcoming Monday.

When I got to work on Monday morning at 7:30am, I called the doctor's office and left a message for an immediate call back. At 10am, no one had called me, so I called again. I was loud and rude, and I told the girl who ran the office about the lump and that I wanted an appointment the next day since I knew the doctor was only in on Tuesday. To my dismay, I was told that the doctor was on vacation and it would be the following Tuesday—a full week away until the doctor could see me! I was furious and wanted to know if there was anyone else I could see. She transferred me to my least favorite nurse. I tried to be calm and explained what was going on.

"You have a CT Scan scheduled on Friday. Go to that. Get your blood drawn, and next week the doctor will see you. There is nothing he can do without the scan and the blood work anyways"

I was furious *"Fine!!"* I hung up.

I went about the next week in a fog. We were supposed to take a family vacation, the first ever in the ten years I had known Chris, both kids and Chris's mom and dad. I had to call and let my mother-in-law know what was going on, and tell her that I thought we were going to have to cancel if I have to start chemotherapy again. I was shocked that this was back. I thought if I had made it through, that I was done with the cancer.

I went on Friday to the imaging center for my scan. The place was over-crowed as usual, but I was prepared this time and showed up a half hour late after my work day was done. They told me I was late and behind. I would have to hurry, as they handed me the cup to drink. I stood at the desk and sucked down the 32ounce drink in less than a minute, set the cup on the counter, and said:

"Now I'm caught up. Start the clock."

The girl smiled and said, *"Wow, you've done this before."*

"Yes, I have."

I found a seat and a half hour later asked to use the rest room. They escorted me through the doors and to the rest room, and I found my way back to the waiting room. I sat there trying to occupy my mind by emailing Chris at work. Another half hour passed, and a young blonde in a lab coat called my name. I headed with her to the scan room. I was prepared this time with no jewelry; I told the tech that I had had a scan before, how they used a child's dose because it made me sick. Her response:

"I've never heard of that."

I pointed to the cabinet she took the contrast out of instead of the one she had reached into.

"That cabinet is empty."

I got on the table, and she headed for my left side.

"I've got one good vein for that needle." I pointed to it on my right arm.

"My IV pole won't move to your right side. It is too tight because they worked on it today," and she reached for my left arm and put the needle in a vein on the side. She taped the needle in place and lifted my arm in the air. I could feel the needle pulling on my arm.

"That hurts."

Her answer to that was more tape around the IV insertion point.

"Ok listen. Try to get the diaphragm in the picture. That is where the cancer was."

"That type of picture wasn't ordered. I can only do what was ordered." and with that she walked towards the door. I could see her through the window as she sat down. My arm was in the air, and I closed my eyes and tried to relax, knowing it would be over in a couple of minutes. Only the table didn't start to move and no lady's voice started to tell me to take a deep breath and hold it. I opened my eyes. The table was still in the middle of the room. My arm was beginning to ache and I

could feel the contrast moving through my head. I started to feel the nausea rising in me, I turned my head to look and the tech was talking on a cell phone! I yelled:

"Can we get this done?!! My arm is throbbing and I'm going to throw up!!"

"Close your eyes and keep your arm up," was the response. Then I heard the machine start up. The three pictures were taken as I went in and out of the machine. Then, I was lying on the table again with no noise and no movement for a minute or two. I finally heard the door open, and I looked to see her approaching my IV arm. She straightened the arm again and checked the IV.

"We're gonna take another set of pictures. He saw something. Hang tight," and with that she was back through the door and behind glass again. I waited and waited only to turn my head and to see her standing there talking to another girl. I felt myself get angry which at that point was probably a good thing because it made me think of something other than puking. I yelled:

"Finish up or I'm getting off the table!" I saw her turn to look at me through the glass and roll her eyes, the other girl immediately left, and the machine started up again. One more picture and then she came through the door. I could feel the pull when she removed the needle, and I knew something was wrong. I know the tech knew too. She wrapped a bandage around my entire arm tightly. When I say tightly, I mean that my skin was bulging on either side of the bandage, and it was painfully uncomfortable.

"Leave this on for at least an hour," She commented. *"You can get up now."*

I got up and looked at her.

"What did you see?"

"The doctor will talk to you about it."

"So, it's Friday, and you want me to wait until Tuesday at 6pm to see the doctor?! What did you see?"

"Nothing. The doctor will talk to you."

Beyond angry, I left. I thought to myself as I drove home, where are all these compassionate people that everyone talks about and write about in all these books about true life cancer stories I was reading?

Because the longer I was at this facility, the more I realized that except for some of the girls who administered the actual chemotherapy that I wasn't getting that 'warm fuzzy feeling' I felt I deserved at this point. Not to mention my concerns and opinions were being totally disregarded! I felt like I was correct, and the cancer was inching in back in April, now it was the beginning of August, and I knew I was fully engulfed.

I met Chris for dinner, and we talked about what had happened to me. He was thinking that there was nobody who really cared about their job any more. I expressed the doubts I was starting to have about this hospital and its workers. He, on the other hand, had faith in the doctor because he had saved my life. With my drive time home and then to the restaurant, dinner, conversation and the ride back to the house, the tight wrap on my arm had been in place over three hours. She had told me *at least* an hour. It was bothering me; I dressed for bed and removed the bandage. The area where the needle had gone in was severely bruised. As I lay watching TV, trying to wind down and not think about what was on my scan, the area started to form a very large hard bump.

"What the hell? Look at this!" I said to Chris.

He wanted to take me to the emergency room. I opted for the computer first. He researched and so did I. From what I was reading it seems it happens when IV's are not inserted properly and they leak medicines into the surrounding area. I was angry that that stupid tech wouldn't listen to me, and I figured, she had double punctured my vein. That moment was another awaking moment for me. I found a new website which led me to several more, chat rooms and threads for medical issues. I bookmarked all of them and spent the weekend reading and researching about all things cancer and any offshoot I found informative. I started to see what good and bad treatment was and what questions I should be asking of my doctor. It was informative and enlightening.

On Sunday, I sat down and wrote a complaint letter about the tech and the imaging center and the hospital as a whole. I sent it to every person at the corporate office I could find online. I put out a message on social media pages asking if anyone knew a person higher up in the hospital system I was using, but I had no luck. My letter was never met with an answer. I don't know what I expected. However, the consistently rude treatment from my oncology nurse, the inconsiderate conversations while taking care of me, the bad IV, and not listening to me had sent me to a breaking point. Then to top it off there was the comment about *'seen something on the scan'* and then leaving me hanging for four full days. I knew I was coming to a turning point in my own care.

I had the feeling the cancer was back. I felt that my treatment compared to other patients I had read about was sub-par. Yet I still didn't have a handle on what to do to effect change in my own care. I was getting more and more frustrated.

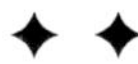

On Tuesday, as I sat in the doctor's office waiting to see him, I had a list of questions and complaints written out. The doctor walked in and there was no open arm hug. He went right to the chair sat down and opened my file.

"Listen. Your numbers jumped up on me."

"To what?"

"596"

"WHAT?!"

"So, we are going to schedule you for two more chemotherapy treatments, and that should take care of it, but first I want you to have that stent placed by the doctor I recommended."

"The tech at the lab said she saw something in the scan."

"Here's the thing. Your number went up, but I want the stent placed, and we will draw blood every two weeks to keep an eye on the number. I think it went up this high because you need the stent. There is no sign of cancer. Your scan is clean."

"What did she see in the scan then?"

"The hydronephrosis which you had before. Don't worry Kim. Your scan shows no cancer."

And with that, he ushered me to the desk to make the arrangements.

"She needs to see Dr. So-and-So right away for a stent and then two rounds," he directed the girls sitting behind the desk. He made some notes in my file folder, handed it to one of the girls, and was on his way.

"Now, don't stress," one of the girls said to me as she reached for a sheet on the printer. She handed me the same name and office info for the doctor I couldn't get a hold of, and a script to have my blood checked again the following Monday.

Angry and confused by everything that happened, I left. I called Chris from the car and told him everything. We were both in shock, and when he got home, we started to talk about the trip and how to handle everything. I took the approach that the pain-in-my-ass nurse had taken in the first place; it was now the first week in August, I will schedule my stent placement after our trip sometime around the 20-25th of the month. Then I will have chemo the Thursday before Labor day and take the Tuesday after Labor Day off. That would give me plenty of time to handle all this, and still go to work.

The next day, I called this new doctor's office several times and finally got an actual person. When I complained about how long it took, they gave me a different number to call to make appointments in the future. The first appointment they had was two and a half weeks away; I thought this to be good because it worked in with what I was planning and our family trip would be fine. I needed that trip. To just have fun and hang out with Chris and the kids. His mom and dad would have a good time, and we would relax and laugh together.

Monday came and I had my blood draw. On Tuesday, I called the office for my number. The girl I always spoke to said,

"Umm… hmm. Just a minute I am going to put you on hold." After several minutes, she came back to the phone.

"Kim, the numbers aren't in the computer yet. I will call you when they are."

I said ok and left it at that. I didn't get a call at all on Tuesday. Preparing to call the office on Wednesday morning my cell phone rang at my desk before I had a chance to call. It was the nurse I detested.

"Hi Kim. I have you set up for chemo on this Friday."

"Wait a minute!" I was shocked and irritated by this woman

again. Her lack of knowledge of what the doctor said irritated me and I needed to walk to a place where I could yell at her. Once in the hallway, I started in.

"This Friday? Well the doctor said I needed to get a stent placed and then chemo. I have an appointment next week with the urologist, then the stent. Set the chemo up for the end of the month the Thursday before Labor Day," I said it with anger and direction. I was sick of this bitch and the way she treated me.

"Why are you going to wait for chemo?"

"Well a year ago you were yelling at me that I was starting too soon! Now I'm starting too late! Make up your damn mind!!"

"Kim your CA125 is 1640. It's higher than before your surgery. You have to start NOW. Get the stent put in this week, and then I will change your chemo till Monday or Tuesday."

"1640? HOW THE HELL DID THAT HAPPEN, IT WAS JUST IN THE 500s!!" At that moment, I realized it was a number that was higher than post-surgery and the 'hit me twice' with chemo wasn't going to work. *"Fine,"* I continued. *"I'll keep the Friday chemo and get the stent after my two treatments."*

"You can't do that! You could go into kidney failure!"

"What the hell do you want me to do?! It's the urologist YOUR office recommended, and I can't get in to see him for over a week!!"

"I know. They should take cancer patients first. I don't know why they don't." It was the first time I heard any compassion in this woman's voice, and I used the opportunity to pounce.

"Can't you call there and ask them to fit me in sooner?"

"Yes, I can do that. I will call you after I do. Don't worry or stress out. It makes things worse."

"Thank you."

I waited all day, no call. I called her back right before 5pm, and she said she hadn't gotten a chance to call, but she would. This was going remarkably bad, and I was watching my life now slip away from me for the second time in a year. It irritated me that I had no control over appointments. That all the things that kept me from going to the doctor for all these years were no better, in fact it was worse. I was no longer riding out a sinus infection; this was do-or-die type stuff. Don't worry. Don't stress. Yet this number of mine was rising rapidly and there was nothing that I could do to stop it. Like the bus in the movie *Speed,* out of control and heading for the end of the pavement.

I had no one to vent to besides Chris because of my decision to keep everything quiet. I bitched a little to my mother-in-law, but there was nothing bitching could even do. I felt like I couldn't fix any of this. I prayed that the doctor was right and that the number was going up because I needed a stent.

I spent the entire night online looking at all these new medical sites I had found and the threads and chat rooms. I signed into one and for the first time asked a question, not of doctors, but of people going through cancer treatments. I typed,

"Hi, my name is Kim, Dx Ovarian Cancer 3b, 6 rounds of carbo/taxol, 7 months of remission, CA125 posting at 1600+ doctor says I need a stent… help? Can the CA125 post that high for a stent?"

I received four responses, and they were all bad news for me. *"Probably not. That is an awfully high number. We'll be praying for you. Keep us posted."* They all had the same thing to say. I was devastated, and still angry that the stupid nurse hadn't done what she said she would do.

On Thursday morning, going on two days with no sleep, I went to work like nothing was wrong. I walked into the bathroom before going to my desk. As I set my purse and lunch box on the vanity surrounding the sink, I looked into the mirror and saw it; the redness was back in my eyes; my skin tone was shallow like I needed more makeup. And the glands, I felt my neck, they were still swollen, not as large as they were, but not normal either. I knew it was back. I didn't care what the scan said. It was hiding somewhere else they couldn't see. Higher up in my body, I was sure of it.

My entire life I had been blessed with this sixth sense. I knew things, about other people, not everyone, but some. I would come in contact with people and 'just know' things. I never knew why, but it was a gift from God I was told early on. My mother had an intuition about things, and so did my youngest sister. I would read Tarot cards from time to time for friends, freaking them out when I could tell them things. It was strange because the cards were a crutch to make others feel better. I didn't really need them. I knew many times, in advance when things were going to happen to me. And yet, through this whole experience, I had ignored every sign. Every little feeling I had, I had dropped the ball on myself, wishing everything would go away. It became clear that this was all going to be part of me for the rest of my days. I also had to learn how to cope with it and trust what I knew in my gut. How I would relay that to medical staff was, at this point, beyond my abilities. I mean, you can't walk into a doctor's office and say, *"hey, I read my own palm and I think that..."* or better yet, *"I had a vision in my dream..."*

My thoughts were broken by my cell phone ringing. I looked at the ID, it was the doctor's office. I tried to be pleasant and upbeat.

"Hello."

"Kim I got you an appointment with the urologist and told them that this needed to be done ASAP. As soon as you go there and get your surgery date, call me back, and I will get you the chemo date immediately following that surgery." She sounded more pleasant than she ever had. I think because I was now at her mercy and needed her to do this scheduling for me.

"I will. Thanks." I hung up. I noted that there was no apology for not calling me back yesterday like she said. It was one more day to check off with the cancer going untreated.

I went to my desk and pulled the small calendar out of my purse to look at the date I had been given to see the urologist. It was the day we were supposed to be leaving to head out on vacation. I went online and cancelled our hotel reservations, and emailed my mother-in-law to let her know. She cancelled the kennel for her dog and her reservations also.

I was lucky in the fact that Chris and I already had the next several days off work, so I didn't have to let anyone know what was going to take place. That night, I went home and looked at all the stuff I had set out to get ready to pack. I had even broken down and cheap old me spent$112 on a Fossil purse that I wanted to buy for our wedding in Vegas and never did. We were very tight on money and our family trip was mostly being financed by my always helpful relatives. For me to buy something so frivolous was not in my nature during times with money issues.

I felt I had made decent money all through my adult working life. In fact, I had started babysitting before and after school for the couple that lived across the street when I was only eleven years old. I had always made money and was able to buy whatever I wanted and had taken full advantage of that. Expensive shoes, other accessories and clothes—I had so many clothes! When Chris and I moved in together, my condo had three full closets, plus a cedar closet in the basement, and eighteen thirty-gallon plastic tubs full. I felt I had lived that lifestyle and I was done. It was way more important to pay my medical, utility and house payments then spend on something like a purse. Yet, Chris insisted. We made the long drive to a more upscale mall about thirty miles from our home—our local mall didn't carry upscale anything. I looked for the purse and found it. I admired the soft leather, and Chris talked me into getting it. He said I deserved it for all I had been through. I made the purchase, and couldn't wait to use it on vacation. Now, it sat on the edge of my dresser mocking me—*told you so; you can't spend like this anymore; who do you think you are?*

"It will be ok. Let me help you put all this away, and then I'll call the kids and tell them," Chris said behind me.

I started to cry. *"No, that's ok. We will still pick them up and just do some fun things around here together. No need to wreck their vacation."*

"It will be ok." He hugged me tight and we sat down on the couch together and watched movies for the rest of the night. I had my computer on my lap and while I was watching the movies, I kept looking up things and reading threads of questions and answers for all kinds of cancer. I had been feeling through this whole thing that I was at the mercy of the doctors and nurses and what they said and, like I said before, never getting that warm-fuzzy-feeling people were talking about when it came to medical professionals. This setback was bothering me. They told me not to worry, and I knew that the CA125 was in no way a definitive test and the doctor said… This doctor also had said a year ago that he thought it was a false positive, and he was wrong. I was beginning to doubt my doctor. That is never a good thing.

CHAPTER TWENTY-FOUR
THE PLANNED BECOME SPONTANEOUS

Friday was supposed to be the day we picked up the kids. They stayed at our house and then early the next day we were all going to head out, packed into Chris's parents SUV. Instead, we were heading to the urologist's office. I was thankful that finally someone at the office had stepped up and helped me get this appointment. I was disappointed that even though he was a doctor in the same healthcare system as the oncologist, I had to have Chris's mom and then Chris run around and get all kinds of test results for the doctor to review. Why couldn't his staff request this stuff? Another inconvenience. I had been given an early morning appointment, and for that, I was grateful. When we opened the door to the office suite at the end of a long hallway, I noticed most of the chairs were full. It was a room of men my dad's age and their wives. I was the youngest, and I thought, the only female patient. There were forms and I assumed I was in for a long wait with all the people in front of me. However, the people were called quickly and left quickly after being seen. I realized there was more than one doctor seeing patients behind the large door. I got called after only a thirty minute wait, and Chris came in with me.

My vitals were taken by a nice girl, and she had me pee in a cup. For the first time ever, someone actually explained the method to using those little cups and how to sanitize yourself and how not to corrupt the sample. I never knew those things and wondered if my samples on all those other exams I had had over the years were even tested. I thought back to the urgent care visit about two months before my first gland swelling incident. I thought I had a urinary tract infection. The doctor had me pee in a cup and afterwards asked if diabetes ran in my family I said no, and he said, *"Then you have a urinary tract infection."* I thought it was odd at the time, but never questioned it. The doctor's didn't know me, and I barely knew myself. I think that if whatever was found in my urine at that point was explored more, (like if I had the same doctor for many years, and the sample was given without contamination) they might have discovered the start of the cancer at that moment.

The doctor came in, introduced himself, and asked for a brief background, and I filled him in. He showed me a picture on the wall of a male's kidney and bladder and joked when pointing to it, *"This is a picture of a boy."* I laughed when he said it and replied, *"The penis was a give-away."* He smiled at me and explained in lay-men's terms what a stent was, what kinds of stents they had and how he would place it in the body. Then, he went on to tell me:

"Normally we do these downstairs, next to the imaging center in the out-patient facility, but I'm going to do yours across the street in the main hospital because I want to get a good picture, and we don't know if there is a blockage. The stents go from very soft flexible plastic to pretty stiff. The stiffer we have to use, the more discomfort you might have, but if by some chance I can't push anything through, like if cancer is blocking something, then we check you into the hospital and the next day we cut into your side and go in that way. So, I want to be over there already in case that happens. Do you understand?"

I nodded yes and at that moment The Other was moving from his seat to the floor. He thought he was going to pass out again. The doctor looked at him on the floor and joked:

"You do know it's her going through this right?"

Chris said, *" Yes, but the technical talk makes me a little..."* He let his voice trail off.

The doctor redirected his attention to me.

"Are you on chemo now?"

"No, last time was Jan 3, but they want to start me again ASAP, so I need to get this done." Knowing he had my scan because I had brought it in and gave it to the girl at the desk, I also interjected, *"You've seen my scan. The oncologist said it was clear. So, do you see a blockage?"*

"We won't know till we get in there."

I was getting conflicting stories now. My oncologist said the tube was extended, and his drawing reflected what I was thinking, a stretched out tube. This doctor was saying blockage, a totally different thing.

"Is there a blockage on the scan?" I said remembering what the last tech said about 'seeing something.'

"I don't know. I'll take my own pictures."

Then I knew he didn't even look at the CT-Scan, which I thought odd because when I was making the appointment, before the nurse stepped in to move it up, the girl on the phone insisted that I would need a CT-Scan before the appointment and wanted to make an appointment for me. I said I already had had two this year, and they should be in my file. That's when she insisted I go get them and bring them along, hence sending my poor mother-in-law on a mad dash to get the information! I don't know why if the doctor didn't even look at them.

I repeated back to the doctor everything he had said and then I asked about side-effects of the stent.

"Be honest. I'm tired of getting all these surprise side-effects with all this cancer stuff. Just tell me the truth."

He laughed again and said, *"Okay. First where is your desk at work in relation to the bathroom? How many feet? You work at a desk right?"* He asked in a double check kind of way.

"Out of the office. Maybe five, six hundred feet."

"You need to be closer."

"I can't, I have one of the closest desks." Which was true.

"Well, then you should wear a little pad or adult diaper. When you have to go, you have to go. Don't wait run! Also, if you do a lot of work, yard work, housework, exercise, any type of movement, you will see a little blood in the urine. Don't call the office. Don't panic; that's normal. And depending on what kind of stent, you might have a little pain."

"That's all *of it?"*

"That's it."

"Okay. How quick can we do this?"

"I talked to your doctor, and he said right away. So I will have my girls schedule you at the beginning of next week, probably Wednesday."

That wasn't the beginning of the week, but it fell on my vacation days so I was good.

"How soon after that can I have chemo?"

"I probably wouldn't do it the day after. You could if you want to but it's probably best to wait an extra day."

"Are you going to put me out?"

"Oh yeah. Not like for a big surgery, but you won't know what's going on."

He asked if I had any other questions and then headed out, telling me I could set everything up at the front desk.

We headed up there and waited until the chart arrived; they of course collected the co-pay and said that I would be called for scheduling. They were running at about two and a half weeks.

"No," I said firmly. *"I already talked the Doctor. I have to start chemotherapy. He said the beginning of next week."* I wanted an answer now before I left. This seemed like it was heading in a bad direction. She asked for help from another girl.

"Yes right here. He's noted to set this up, with a date. That's next Wednesday." Then, she turned to look at me *"Someone will call you from scheduling. I'm thinking by 5pm to set this up."*

"It's marked for across the street, right?"

"Yes it is." She looked at the other girl. *"Call there to make sure they put this at the top of the list."* The first girl said ok, and they both told me to have a nice day and enjoy the weekend.

In the car on the way home, Chris asked if I wanted to grab some lunch before we picked up the kids. I said I wanted to go home and pee first and then yes. I thought to myself that I sure hoped that this need to pee every thirty minutes or so would go away with this surgery. Frequent urination is one of the signs of ovarian cancer, and I was the queen. However, that need did not vanish after the first surgery or the following chemotherapy treatments. I still had to go as much as I ever had. As soon as we walked in the door the phone rang, it was scheduling—I was all set for Wednesday and to call the night before for exact times and instructions.

I looked at Chris when I got off the phone *"Let's still go with the kids for a shorter amount of time."*

"What?!" he said with his retentive panic setting in.

"Sure, it's only 10:30 right now. We'll pick up the kids and go. Instead

of our plan to drive to Mackinaw City early on Saturday, we'll get the kids like around one and head to Frankenmuth, spend the night there, stop at The Christmas Store and walk around the city, then tomorrow drive to Mackinaw, stop at the Cross and some tourist spots, spend Saturday night around the City; on Sunday, we'll go to the island, and drive home on Monday. Two days shorter, but we'll cut out the Falls and the Upper Peninsula. We can do this! Call your mom now!"

Chris grabbed the phone, and I started packing the suitcases. His mom and dad decided not to go because I had jumped the gun and that forced them to cancel the kennel for their pets, so we were on our own. I called a hotel in Frankenmuth and made reservations and then called the Hotel in Mackinaw City that I had canceled my reservation for yesterday. I explained my story and asked if I could still get a room. The city was busy in the summer and I hoped that I could get it back. They were booked, my heart sank. This might put a crimp in my little plan. The girl was very nice and said that they had a sister property. It was farther down the road but still on the water and very nice, and she showed openings. Then she gave me the number, and I had a reservation! I was thrilled.

I ran around the house, throwing everything together. I texted the kids that their dad was picking them up early, and Chris ran out to get them while I finished up the packing. If there is one thing cancer does teach you—it is to 'live in the moment.' The future is incredibly uncertain with all types of cancers, so when an opportunity arises, you have to move. The planning that Chris and I did in the past was out the window. Now we had to run in the moment.

When the kids walked in all smiles, I said we were changing plans, no grandma and grandpa, and we are leaving now, not tomorrow. Then, came the hard part I had to tell them both why and that the cancer was back.

I could see the sadness in both of their faces, especially Hunter. My step daughter, Kaitlin spoke up first:

"But you're gonna be alright? Right?"

Chris said, *"Oh course she is, but right now, and this weekend, we are gonna think about our trip and have fun!"*

And we did. The kids took everything out to the car, and we

were off, with my new purse hanging off my shoulder. I felt great, and I was happy. We spent four glorious days with these remarkable Little Ones, and I loved every minute of it. We took them to all the places my parents had taken me when I was growing up. I had been to these places dozens of times but they all seemed new and vibrant sharing them with the kids.

On the ride home on Monday everyone was quiet. The last day of vacation is always hard. They slept in the back seat on and off, and the music played off The Other's mp3 player. I was left alone with my thoughts.

What if this was it? The last trip with my family, the last time we'll all be together like this. The reality was coming back into my thoughts, having pushed all of it aside for a few wonderful days. I wish I could skip all the appointments like I used to in my twenties when my schedule didn't work out. Didn't call to cancel; didn't show up. Nobody noticed; nobody cared.

I knew that Wednesday was a short time away, and it was all coming back…Every lousy, crappy thing that happens during chemotherapy.

Living here, sick and tired, sick of being sick, tired of being depressed. They don't tell you these things when you start the chemo. Then you are stuck. Your family and friends all expect you to fight, when deep inside you want to throw in the towel."

- Michelle
6 year colon cancer survivor- 4 rounds of chemotherapy

CHAPTER TWENTY-FIVE
IT'S ALL ABOUT THE PEE

We showed up for my outpatient surgery right on time. We were in the same hospital, but sent this time to a different area. It was small room with low ceilings, very dingy. The lady behind the reception counter was a senior, and her badge said volunteer. She didn't have much to say in the way of instructions when we were sent to her other than:

"Have a seat."

We waited together. Chris tried to take my mind off things and be funny. Over the last couple of days, I had gotten up the nerve to tell Chris that I felt when he passed out or his mom cried during a doctor's visit that the focus came off me and on to the two of them. I wanted him to come with me every time, but if he wasn't feeling strong enough, I could totally understand him staying in the waiting room. He understood, and we came to an agreement on how to handle things in the future. I liked the fact that this urologist wasn't swayed by Chris's getting light-headed; it showed me focus on his part. A focus on me. I am sure the difference between being an urologist and an oncologist is that there is much more bad news with the latter, and I am sure people get emotional. I was tired of the emotional. I wanted to go back to cold hard facts only.

After about a half an hour, a nurse finally came and called my name. There was no introduction or name tags, no board, no pleasantries like last time. I followed her back. The start was the same, questions, changing clothing into hospital garb. The nurse listened to my whole story and asked a ton of questions. I got the feeling she was stalling for time. Finally, a second nurse came in, and she was introduced as my pre-op nurse; she apologized for being late, and the first nurse caught her up. She started an IV in the top of my hand, even though I once again mentioned the port, which she wasn't trained to use either, and she sat down, put on her glasses, and took her time putting in the needle. She asked if she could bring anyone back. I told her Chris, and she went and got him. He sat with me for quite a while before my doctor showed up, he said,

"You doing okay?"

"Yes."

"Ok, I got one in front of you, and then they'll come and get you, ok?!" With that he tapped my leg down by my shin in a very comforting, confident manner and he left.

Chris and I sat and talked as the medicine kicked in and I found myself relaxing. I hated that they made you lay back. I wanted a more upright position. I didn't like lying on my back.

After almost an hour, a male nurse came in, asked the same questions the anesthesiologist asked for the last surgery, and he said it would only be a few more minutes. He said he worked with my doctor directly, then asked if I needed something. I said:

"I really have to go to the bathroom."

"Don't worry. They are going to put a catheter in you once you are under, we will get that all out."

"I don't want to pee all over the doctor."

He laughed, "You wouldn't be the first, and the staff thinks it's funny when that happens."

"Ok but seriously I've been here over three hours. I'm an old woman. I have to pee."

"Alright, they don't like you walking around with all that medicine in you, so let me help you."

He disconnected the IV from the pole. I had learned how to navigate dragging the pole, but he made it so much easier. He wrapped a blanked around me, and made sure I got to the bathroom okay and then hooked me back up.

"I feel so much better. Thank you."

"No Problem." And with that, Chris had to go back to the waiting room.

Three people wheeled me into the surgical room. It was different this time, and I was set next to a tall upright white machine. I heard the male nurse say:

"I will talk to you when you wake up."

And with that, I was in my dreamless sleep like the last surgery. The next thing I actually felt was the gurney I was laying on being rolled down a hall, and walking next to me was the male nurse. I thought that it must be easier remembering all the men in the office to have a male nurse for their surgeries.

"Hey Kim! You did great!" he shouted walking alongside the gurney.

"Did they get the stent in?"

"Yep, everything went great"

"Which kind the flexible one or the stiff one?" I remembered the doctor showing me the tube with its two little coiled ends.

"I'll let the doctor talk to you about all that."

"Okay. Hey, I really need to pee again, badly!" I was remembering what the doctor said about the stent and having to pee and to head to the bathroom right away.

"Don't worry that's from the surgery it will go away soon. You have nothing left in your bladder we have a catheter in."

"But it really feels like I have to go."

"Don't you worry yourself about that. It will be okay." He took my hand in his and said, *"I wish you the best of luck with all your treatments. You hang in there and be strong."* FINALLY! Someone who took it upon themselves to read my chart! That made me happy.

He left, and the other two people wheeled me into a large curtained room. It was darker than the last time as some of the florescent lights above were burned out, and there was only one stand that seemed to have every monitor I needed attached to it. Chris came in, and they found him a chair to sit in.

The nurse wanted me to partially sit up and eat some graham crackers and juice. I asked for cranberry.

"Oh look! Yay! It's the chemo-lab diet." I remarked to Chris

Having sat through one of my chemos, he knew as I had sent him for these tasty *insert sarcasm* treats many times. I told the nurse monitoring me that I had to pee. She said,

"No you don't. It's from the surgery." She was nice, but I told Chris

it really feels like I have to pee. There was an aide in the general area; I saw her coming and going, bringing in wheelchairs and wheeling people out. She checked on most of the patients on her turns back to pick up a new person to escort out. She politely asked if I needed anything, and she had stuck her head in as the nurse was saying that I don't have to go. Unfortunately, trying to get the aide to help me find a restroom was also going to be out of the question.

After about ninety minutes, with each fifteen minutes them raising my bed up a little higher until I was fully upright and then sitting in the chair next to the bed, the nurse told me I could get dressed, and she disconnected the IV. When she did that, she held the cotton pad on the spot the needle had been inserted on. I had only seen one other lab tech do that on a blood draw, and I thought that lady did it because we were talking, and she didn't want to turn away to get a bandage. While she stood there holding my hand tightly between her thumb and forefinger, I told her about the incident with the CT tech.

She said, *"That's why I am applying pressure. I felt the vein pull when I took the needle out. It was a bad puncture. You have to apply pressure right away and hold it or you can have problems like that. How big did it get?"*

"Like half a golf ball on my arm."

"See, that's just sloppy. I'm going to wrap this really tight too. Leave it on till tomorrow if you can stand it. The longer the better."

"Ok."

Then, I got dressed. Chris helped me, and I started talking in a hushed tone.

"Some of these nurses know more than others. I'm gonna start asking them a lot more questions. See that tech did screw up! I should sue. I'm sick of people not doing their jobs, and after I told her exactly what I needed!"

He agreed and when I was fully dressed and I was sitting back in the chair he opened up the front of the curtain. The young aide appeared with a wheelchair. The nurse had me sign some forms and gave me instructions for the day.

"Lots and lots of water. Flush all that out okay?! And make sure you eat when you get home. Good luck to you."

The aide pushed me out of the recovery area, and as soon as we were clear of the nurses she whispered in my ear:

"Do you want to use the ladies room?"

"YES!"

"Okay. Hang out till I get you outta here."

We went through the door and around a corner. She pushed me up to the entrance of the bathroom.

"Be careful. If you need me to come in there and help you, just holler ok? I'll be right outside the door."

I went in thankful that it was a single with handicap grab bars. My right hand was bandaged, and I was very wobbly, but I sat down and peed better than I had in years! It felt great. I turned around to look. There was a bit of blood, but not a lot.

I went back out to the wheelchair.

"Was there a lot of blood?" The aide asked.

"No, surprisingly not, but there was a lot of pee!"

She laughed. *"They are used to doing that surgery on men. Women are different. We have to pee all the time! I know I do."* She finished wheeling me out to the parking lot, and Chris helped me to the car.

The rest of the day Chris waited on me, and I relaxed and slept on and off. By the next day, I woke up and felt great. As the week progressed, I noticed I could sleep through the night without getting up to pee, and I didn't have to pee every hour. In fact, for the first time in my life, even with upping my water consumption to two quarts a day like they recommended on line, I was only visiting the bathroom a few times a day, not a dozen like before. There was no urgency, no accidents, no leaking, no pain, and no blood.

On my check-up about a month later, I joked and said, *"I should have had this put in years ago! I finally feel like I don't have to go to the bathroom 24/7!"*

CHAPTER TWENTY-SIX

ARE YOU OUT OF YOUR MIND?

I had called my least favorite oncology nurse the day before my surgery. She scheduled me for the following Monday, five short days away, and the day I was supposed to return from vacation. I ended up working from home on Thursday and Friday following the surgery to save up the vacation days. I also had to come clean with work. There was no way I could do this I had decided, and why would I want to. I told them about the stent and the fact that I needed two more chemo treatments. I said I would take vacation days for the treatment, work from home for the following week, and then be back in the office. So I really wasn't missing anything. They seemed fine with it, and, it was only going to be two treatments, at least that's what the doctor said.

When I was talking to the nurse she was reviewing what they gave me last time. Then, she said she was going to change one of my anti-nausea meds, I asked why and she said, *"You don't need to be on all this medicine."*

"I get very sick. Not only do I need it, but I will need a script for seven days' worth of pill Zofran and a stool softener and Motrin 600."

"I don't think you need all of that."

"I took it last time, and I WANT it again."

"Alright fine, but the insurance company is not going to give you more than twenty Zofran pills a month."

"They did last time."

"Oh, ok."

I thought 'great, now she's an expert on my insurance!' I continued to speak,

"Also, the Compazine makes me nuts in the head. It puts me into a coma, I want something else."

"Nuts in the head? I don't think so."

"I am telling you – it makes me weird, doped up. I don't want to feel like that. You said there were hundreds of anti-nausea medicines. I want a different one!"

I wasn't taking any crap this time. I didn't care which pharmaceutical rep was pushing which drug. I wanted what was best for me. If that meant they had to do a little research, *you know their jobs,* then so be it…

"Well, there's not hundreds." She corrected me, as if I didn't hear her right a year ago.

"That's what YOU told me! Now prescribe something different!"

"Okay, I will."

She said I was all set for 8 am and gave me a day to stop by and get my scripts and give blood. Then she asked,

"Do you still have your port in?"

"Yes."

"Oh good. We usually take those out at six months."

I wanted to say, yeah the smart, nice nurse who administers my chemo warned me. It is a good thing nobody had suggested I do that in June. Maybe my suspicions made them antsy.

I felt that I was finally starting to speak up more. I was sick to death of feeling like shit, and I wanted them to do something about it even if I had to pull Mean Kim out of the closet.

'Mean Kim' was a nickname I was given. She was the person I was back in my twenties and thirties: a say-anything, step-on-anyone-to-get-what-I-wanted-or-needed, a young, arrogant version of me. I had no other ambition than to work, make money, and use that money to buy what I wanted and travel where I wanted to. I didn't take shit from anyone, and I didn't care who I hurt to benefit myself.

In a self-realization moment not long after my first marriage of nine years ended in 1999, I realized Mean Kim was actually Unhappy Kim. I started to fix all the unhappiness in my life and Mean Kim went into a closet, and she very seldom had to show her head again. I pulled her out on purpose when I felt someone I loved was being taken advantage of. But I never again used her to get what I wanted out of life, instead choosing to live in a happier place.

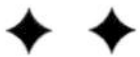

I went to the hospital that Friday, got my scripts filled there, and headed over to the lab. I also had to talk to the wonderful dietician who was teaching the bariatric class I had started attending. I had learned more about health, dieting and nutrition in the four weeks with her than my whole life of dieting, listening to TV-show doctors, and reading magazine articles. There was so much I had been doing wrong in following all these idiots and fad dieting. I loved all the people in my class, and I was really sorry to have to leave it. I explained it all to her, and she was very sympathetic and said I could rejoin another class if I wanted to after my two chemo treatments.

When I picked up the pills. the pharmacy only gave me twenty instead of thirty, I asked why. She said that was all my insurance would cover.

"Bullshit! They covered thirty pills last time!"

"Sorry, there's nothing I can do."

I realized that I had my scripts filled at a chain drugstore last time. There was no refill on the bottle, and I had a few pills left from last time, so I made a note to not get any more scripts filled at the hospital. When I got home, I looked at the pill. They didn't look like my other Zofran pills. They were marquee-shaped, like the diamond, and my other ones were round. This worried me. Also I used to get the entire white plastic bottle, and this time they had been counted into the standard orange bottle. More and more, this hospital wasn't sitting right with me. It seemed at every turn there was an issue or worse… a mistake being made.

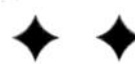

Monday came and Sue and I made our regular trek to the cancer center in the hospital. Once I checked in, they sent me back to my usual private room. The nurse I liked came in and said that my chemo was the same, but they ordered different medicines for side effects. I wasn't happy about this and neither was she. One of the things that was missing was the Aloxi, which was the multi-day, time release anti-nausea med. I asked what the difference was going to be

she said:

"These other ones are pills. You have to take them like clockwork. You get very sick, I would think they would want to add this extra little push for a few days." But she qualified her statement and said, *"but they know what they're doing it will be fine."*

I went through the treatment and I didn't have my list from before but I felt like something else had been eliminated. With the treatment ending about forty-five minutes early, I knew I was right.

I went home and even on the drive I felt sick. I usually didn't start getting really sick until two days later—that's when the worst of it kicked in. I also had another problem. I couldn't drink water. It tasted bad, and with the stent I knew I had to. I drank a lot of other beverages but I knew not having enough water was going to be bad. My taste buds were changing with this one new dose of chemotherapy.

I had my routine with the pills. For the ones at night, I would have Chris make me a bowl of cereal, so I wasn't taking anything on an empty stomach. On the second night, I ate the cereal, took the pill and no more than three minutes later ran to the bathroom to vomit. I watched all the cereal come back up, as I felt the pee pour down my leg and soak my pajamas. I started to cry as Chris stood in the doorway and asked if I needed help.

"Is Hunter in his room?"

"Yep, upstairs sound asleep. I checked"

I had been trying to keep all these terrible side effects from him; I was successful for the most part.

"I need pajamas," I said through my tears, he laid them out on the bed, and I started to clean up my mess… Again.

"Beez, just leave it. I'll clean it up. That's what I'm here for. Leave those pajamas in there."

I took off my pee-soaked pajama's and left them on the floor, grabbed a towel out of the closet, and dried off and put on the clean pajama's The Other had put out for me. Then, I laid in bed sick to my stomach crying. I knew things would only get worse. I wasn't positive, but I thought I might have thrown up the pill I just took. Unsure of what to do, I grabbed another one and swallowed it. I watched Chris cleaning up the bathroom as I lay on the bed. He was such a good man. I couldn't believe he was doing all this. He came in the bedroom and sat next to me.

"You ok?" He said rubbing my forehead.

"No, I can't go through this again, and why am I throwing up after two days? That stupid nurse thinks she knows everything. I know she changed the doctor's instructions. I hate her!"

"It's ok. Forget her. We'll sue her later. I just need you to focus and get well."

"Why do you take such good care of me?"

"Because you would do it for me, and I need you here for a long time. Don't worry about that kind of stuff. I'm good at cleaning."

He was, and I appreciated that. I thought about all the men I had dated in my life; none of them would have stuck it out like this, made it all about me and not about them, put up with me and clean up this stuff. It was embarrassing to have to walk past the person you love, the one you always tried to look your best for, tried to be sexy for. Now, I walked from room to room, huge scar running from my pelvic bone past my belly button covered in urine, no hair, no eyelashes, and no eyebrows. I was not a person that anyone would be physically attracted to, and yet this man still liked to hug me, lie on the couch together, and kiss me. He still wanted to be together as a couple whenever I felt up to it. I felt I was letting him down in so many ways.

"Hey! Are you listening to me?" He knocked me out of my train of thought, *"You would take care of me right?"* and he smiled.

I smiled back *"Hell no! Vomit makes me puke!"*

He laughed, *"Then we would be puking together – in buckets!"*

I was laughing now instead of crying *"Well, then yeah, I would clean up the bathroom, but you would clean up the puke"*

"Well as long as you change my crappy adult diaper, I'll clean up the puke."

"Ok, it's a deal."

Our sick sense of humor had gotten me through what would have been a horrible moment. He sat there even though he had to work in the morning and rubbed my forehead till I fell asleep. The alarm went off for the next pill four hours later, and he got up and made me a bagel and made sure I took the pill and then went back to sleep again. Amazing.

I ended up being sick for seven straight days. I was supposed to be back at work on Tuesday, and on Monday night I knew I couldn't. I hadn't had my big shit blowout yet, the one that usually came on Sunday night. I was afraid it would happen at work. I had a new way to help me try and poop regularly; my friend Jenn had a soup she made—it was cabbage based and full of fibrous veggies. I was eating a small bowl every day, and I was able to go a little bit everyday but not enough. I knew the backup was going to come about soon. I had taken my last Zofran on Saturday and nothing yet. Apple cider, the stool softeners, trying to clear this all in time for work on Tuesday; I sucked it up and emailed the HR girl that I wasn't going to make it back to the office until Wednesday. Thank goodness I did, because at 8:30 am, which would have put me at the office for over an hour the gas pains started. I knew it was coming. By 9 am, I was in the bathroom. It was coming out in waves. I was thankful not to be puking, but it smelled. I couldn't even imagine having to do this at work. For the next four hours, round after round of the most painful, burning diarrhea; how in the hell am I going to work like this?

I sat down. I needed to get our bills down to where we could live without my salary. I looked at our house payment. We were ten years into a thirty year loan on our house, but I had put down a sizeable down payment. I went online and found a mortgage calculator. My interest rate was 6.38% and the new rates were down around 3.5%. I had another problem: we needed a second toilet. It was hard for people to ask to use the bathroom making sure I didn't have to go in and they had enough time to shower or shave. The Little One was getting older and even though he didn't seem to care, I didn't like him having to do that. I knew I could get my brother-in-law Ken to help Chris put a bathroom in the basement, but I wasn't sure how I was going to get the money to pay for it. There was a considerable savings monthly on the house payment with a new interest rate. I figured I could go before the tax tribunal and ask for a reassessment for property taxes. I was still coming up about a twelve hundred a month short; I still needed to bring in that much money. We were down to the bare essentials. We splurged on nothing. It was the extra medical bills and the cost of gas-every time it went over $3 a gallon with Chris's long ride to work. I looked on line to see if there were any cheap homes or apartments close to his work, thinking that would save us hundreds in gas money, but it was more money than what I owed on the house we were in. I picked up the phone and called the very large bank that held my mortgage.

Now let me say this. Thanks to my friends and family, I never missed a mortgage payment or was even late. I have held mortgages in my name just under a dozen times as I moved around and bought and sold homes. My credit rating was superior; I protected it, because I thought it would be all I had to rely on going into retirement. I talked to the bank, and they said I was a perfect candidate for the new government sanctioned refi.... Here was the problem, even though I only owed about 82K, my house was estimated to be worth only 72K, I would have to come to the closing with ten grand. If I had ten grand, I'd put in a bathroom and add a garbage disposal to the kitchen along with a dishwasher.

There was only one thing left to do. Move. I'd find a foreclosure, since they were obviously so cheap in my area. Hunter would go to the same school. I would pick a house closer to the high school and then he could walk instead of being driven. I emailed Chris at work and told him my plan. He said

"You want to move during chemo?"

"Oh yeah, I've got it all figured out. We'll get a house cheaper than what we owe, buy it and save on our house payment, plus I'll get the second bath and garbage disposal."

"Whatever you think." I'm reasonably sure he thought I was nuts.

I emailed my real estate lady and asked her if it was possible. She said there were homes out there in the area I wanted with what I wanted, and I said start sending me stuff. I had set the ball in motion.

I went to work the next day, and I knew what was coming. 'The

talk', you need to work-part time from home. Only this time I was ready and had a plan, I said I wanted to do that (words that I never in my life thought I would utter), but I needed my full-time position until I either refinanced or bought something new. I had some things to get in order. My boss agreed to let me stay on full-time for a few more months until I got my life in order. We worked out a salaried part-time position for me where I could work from home and be in the office a couple of days if I felt up to it. I was thrilled with the arrangement, and I knew the time was coming where I would have to resign to myself that my full-time work life was over. With my work life in a good place, I knew we would still be able to handle the insurance co-pays and deductibles as well as all the add-on medical expenses. I felt like a weight had been lifted. I thanked God that this job was sent to me because I knew had I been in hospitality I would have been let go and suing under the Disabilities Act.

With the work end covered, I figured I had about two weeks to get this ball rolling and find a house before the next chemo was going to kick in. We took the weekends and a few hours after work and looked at homes. The problem with me is when it comes to homes after flipping so many of them, I see the 'potential' in every single house. Chris and my real estate agent kept me focused. I hadn't bought a house to flip since before I got sick and the rules of the game of real estate had changed like everything. We were looking for cheap and finished, real close to the high school Hunter would be attending next year. We were running into the same problem however on every house.... leaking basement. We eventually found something, that had a leak we could live with and in about two months' time would be moving.

I loved moving. The house we were in presently was the longest I had lived anywhere except for one of my childhood homes. I was so excited, and every day that I felt good was spent packing up the house. I put out a for 'rent sign' on our current home figuring I could rent it out to cover the mortgage, taxes, and insurance. The calls started coming in and people started filling out applications. It wasn't long before I had three qualified families.

I loved the house I lived in, and I knew what was out there for sale. My house was in far superior shape when it came to the bones. The basement didn't leak; it had new windows, roof, furnace, and air. I also had had the porches redone as well as the patio. When I saw the crap that was out there, mine needed paint, and a kitchen and bath redo because they were dated, but they were functional. I contacted Alison and her fiancé because I knew they were looking and had seen the crap out there. They were interested, I cut my rent, so it would just cover bills with me not making a profit and they moved in hoping to eventually buy the house once they were married in a year or so. I was happy. All my hard work and money spent would be passed on to friends. It gave me one less thing in my life to stress over.

As I started to tell friends my new grandiose plans, my close friend Bob called. Bob and I had spent the better part of ten years as very close friends, talking over dinners and hanging out. He was there dragging my drunk-ass home from the bar after my divorce. Our lives had moved in different directions, but we kept in touch, or should I say as was the case with all my friends, he called me and I was always happy to hear from him. He worked 60+ hours a week and had a very full personal life, needless to say, a busy man. He had started calling me very regularly after every chemo to check on me, and this time was no different. I told him my plan to move again. This guy had physically moved me twice. Never mincing words, he was the Male version of Charlotte. He told me flat out, *"You are a nut and need to get your head examined."* He was right but I went ahead with my plans anyways.

CHAPTER TWENTY-SEVEN
ANOTHER PROBLEM AT THE HOSPITAL

Chemo number two in this second round came up in September; as Sue and I sat down in our usual room, our nurse yelled from the desk:

"So they switched you back to all the old meds, huh?"

"What?!"

"What's listed is everything from your last rounds. That's better. You'll have the Aloxi again. How did you fair last time?"

"Wait, why did they switch it?"

"You didn't call to ask for it to be switched?"

"No."

"I bet I know what happened. They only changed it in the computer for the one month, not continuously. The chemo is the same. It's just the meds for the side effects that are different."

I was furious. I hadn't told anyone about the issues I was having with side-effects on the last treatment. I was going to do that today. It also screamed that no one ever looked at my file from month to month. Did anyone even check the numbers from the blood draws to see if everything was going ok? I bet they never looked at anything! What the hell was going on in this place? I knew it from the first time I talked to that bitch that I didn't like her. My great TV- show-like doctor checked nothing, relying on his nurses for support and information. Furious was probably an understatement at this point.

"Does that happen a lot?"

I never got an answer to that question.

I was whispering to Sue now. I was done with this hospital. It was time for a change. She agreed and vented with me for most of the morning. The office girl showed up with my calendar for labs, an appointment to see the doctor, and a tentative chemo scheduled.

I looked at the calendar and said to her:

"So two treatments wasn't enough?"

"Well, the doctor only ordered two, but I scheduled it just so it's done. We can always cancel it after you see the doctor."

"Fine." I was still seething, and I'm sure my 'fine' came out in a very dismissive manner.

I got home that night and started to think about all the lies I was told, or if not lies, the truth that was omitted, which is right up there with a lie. First, I was lead to believe that if chemo worked, I was good; second, that I would need two more if my numbers did happen to jump up. With the clean scan that the doctor referred to, I really thought these two were precautionary and that once the stent was working I would be good. Wrong again. I was so frustrated, I forgot to ask for my numbers at the hospital, but I couldn't bring myself to call there and talk to anyone in that place.

The next morning I called the big cancer center in my area, the one that was rude to me on the phone, I looked up their TV commercial first and watched and listened closely.

"When the diagnosis is cancer…"

It was subtle wording. They don't diagnosis it. They need to know first. It made more sense. The girl on the phone just couldn't explain that correctly I tried to qualify in my own head. Yet I know I was no longer going to put up with half-assed answers and dismissive tones.

I picked up the phone and called.

"Hi, my name is Kim, and I am currently in chemo for Ovarian Cancer, and I want to switch to your center."

"Okay Kim. I can help you with that."

Sticking with my 'Mean Kim' persona I continued, *"I am not running around and getting records. You will have to do that. I will sign whatever you need. And I want a good doctor, not one that will hold my hand; my husband does that. I want someone who is brutally honest and doesn't hold back, and if you don't have a doctor like that, tell me now. I don't want to hear the word "protocol" or "I have to." I want someone who is going to put me first."*

"Okay, Kim. Why don't you tell me why you want to switch mid-

treatment."

I explained the entire long story and every little detail I could remember. The person on the other end listened, and I could hear them typing on the other end. Every once in a while they would ask me to repeat something.

"So your last infusion was yesterday?"

"Infusion?"

"Your last round of chemotherapy."

"Yes."

"Okay, I would like you to come in on Monday with Doctor So-and-So. Check in at the front desk and they will guide you. I will send you some things in the mail for your first visit."

"What about my records from the other hospital?"

"Do you have an email?"

"Yes."

"I will email you a form. Sign it. Send it back, and I will get all records copied and sent over."

I gave my email and both married and maiden name to assure she'd get everything.

I showed up at this cancer center in the heart of the city. I didn't like the area, it was twice as far, and a much harder drive. It took almost ten minutes just to wait in line for a Valet parking attendant. I wasn't impressed. Everyone in the place moved slow, patients and employees. I remembered the valet parking company from my past jobs again. Those guys ran. The entire shift. Back and forth. The valet attendants here sauntered around with no purpose. I was pleasantly surprised, however, when I got out of the car, how nice everyone was. From the Valet attendants, the security guards inside the door, and the employees I passed; every one of them looked me in the eye and said good morning. I got in line at the front desk and within minutes it was my turn. They gave me a hospital wristband, checked me into the computer and told me to have a seat. Less than five minutes, later someone approached me and said, *"Ms. Henderly can you step over to*

my window." She pointed to the other side of the room where there were several desks with privacy dividers.

She entered all my information into the computer and scanned in the forms I had filled out at home from the mailed packet, including my written list of what I had been through over the past fourteen months. She gave me a folder to keep my paperwork in and called for someone to walk me to my clinic. Unfortunately, the guide I was given barely spoke English and could answer none of my questions as we walked down the halls; I tried to remember where everything was and how to get back to the door, but this place was huge inside. I would later realize that my guide sucked. As I went to this facility more and more, I would hear other people being escorted around by guides. They had answers to a lot of questions and were much easier to understand. But at that moment, I was stuck with this person. So far, this place was 50/50 over the crap I was dealing with. The tour that made no sense ended at the far end of the hall.

She said as we approached,

"All cancer have own clinic. This yours." She motioned me to the desk and gave my name in a thick accent. A pleasant girl told me to have a seat, and I would be called shortly. Sue and I took the last two chairs, and our guide came over to 'explain' the folder the person had given me at the desk. She made no sense pointing out the pen and paper inside, along with other things; her descriptions were garbled and meaningless. She asked if I had any questions and I thought *you couldn't answer them anyways, so who cares.*

Sue asked what I thought of the place. I told her we'll see. The jury's still out. Then, we waited, and waited after forty minutes Sue went to the desk.

"You know she's very sick from chemo. How much longer?"

"Not long, there was an emergency."

Another thirty-five minutes passed and finally they called my name. The young lady however was the aide, she took my vitals, asked a few questions, and sent me back out to the waiting room. I noticed the women in the clinic brought lunches and computers to occupy their time. A mistake I wouldn't make again.

When they called me back into a room, I had been waiting just short of two hours. Luckily the wait in the room wasn't as long. The doctor entered with three other people. He introduced everybody. The ones I paid attention to were the resident and the oncology nurse. He told me his nurse had 99 years of experience and was always reachable and she handed me her card. Page me anytime but give me time to call you back. Sometimes it takes a while. The doctor then said, *"You talk to her in between appointments. You'll see me before each infusion."*

There was that word again—*infusion.*

The doctor was tall and thin and spoke quickly. He was a little hard to understand, but I quickly adapted. My choice to do this alone was for my own benefit. I didn't want to be distracted or have anyone else distract by tears, or anything else. I wanted to be 'Mean Kim,' and I had a list of demands and questions that if these people couldn't answer, I wasn't staying here.

The doctor pushed on without pausing, *"I've read your file; tell me why you want to leave the Great Doctor So and So."* He knew him and didn't find many people who wanted to leave his care. I told him everything. All the hospital errors, and that I didn't like his staff, and that I felt like I wasn't getting the best treatment possible.

He was blunt, and explained first what platinum sensitive was and that he wasn't sure putting me on the same chemo as the first round would work. *"You are right on that border where maybe it works, maybe it doesn't. So next week I want to send you to come back for blood work and another CT scan."* He told me in Europe they didn't rely much on the CA125 but on an actual scan of what was there-inside the body. That made sense. I told him I thought the cancer was back, even though my scan showed clear and told him the symptoms and for how long they had been going on. He listened carefully and the resident took notes. I told him about the CT scans and how I thought they weren't high up enough, and how I thought no one was checking my file month to month and the incident with the medicines changing. I told him I was sick of being sick with the side-effects and about the severe constipation. I laid it all out–about being told that if the first round worked I was lead to believe I was done.

He explained how some doctors think and work. He was extremely blunt about his thoughts on every detail that had happened to me. He was forth right in answering my questions, adding what he thought I needed to know, not running around the answer and avoiding. Most of all, he treated me like I was intelligent, not like I was a helpless person that he needed to hide information from. He didn't necessarily agree that the scan I had gotten was 'clear.' *"Something is going on. You have symptoms and your numbers are high, but a high number could be something else. So we will have another look with our scans. If it looks like the Taxol/Carbo is working, we will keep you on it. If not we will put you on something else."*

After he left, the nurse stayed on to go over what would happen and how chemotherapy worked. You will get your labs once every three weeks; on the same day, you see the doctor and then receive your treatment. I was so glad I didn't have to drive downtown four times a month. I was also glad I would be seeing the doctor all the time, too. This way if something went wrong, I had a doctor to complain to.

My chemo was being moved to every three weeks instead of four. The doctor, in our conversation, said I looked healthy and could handle it. It was a matter of opinion whether you were treated once every three or once every four weeks, and that nobody really knows what works. He explained that it wasn't too long ago when they treated thirteen times no matter what, and in those days sometimes the treatment and not the cancer caused death. I agreed I would try every three weeks hoping that we could knock this out quicker, and with my new work schedule, I wouldn't have to worry about the days off. I was a little concerned about moving and not having that extra week of feeling half-way decent, but I didn't think I'd need too many treatments either.

My nurse asked me about my nausea meds. I told her what they were giving me and that they barely kept it under control. She said they didn't use Aloxi and I told her how bad I had it without it. They were going to get me approval for an anti-nausea medicine called Emend instead. She walked me over to *Infusion Scheduling* where I asked her about scripts. She wrote it for the Motrin 600, Zofran, and a steroid to go with the Emend. She said to page her on Thursday for the CT-Scan results. I thanked her and she headed back to the clinic; leaving me to wait for an infusion scheduler.

I had been looking around since I got here. What I noticed most was the sheer number of people here. Hundreds and hundreds, and all this place did was cancer. Every race, male and female, young and old, cancer didn't care who you are, rich or poor, every type of person was represented. I remembered back to my first phone call here. Other than the rudeness what stuck out from that conversation was *"what type of insurance do you have?"* That really is the bottom line-isn't it? Hundreds and hundreds of people walked around here, or were being wheeled around. They all couldn't be funded by private insurance? Could they? No wonder our system was broke. I also wondered what type of pro-bono work this hospital does. I did know this: that the minute they got my name last year, I was on their fundraising list and was already getting brochures to donate.

It wasn't but a few minutes and I was next at the "infusion scheduling" window. I had put two and two together by now and realized that infusion and chemotherapy were the exact same thing. Why this cancer hospital called it infusion instead of what it was ... chemotherapy... was unknown to me. I could only think that some suit, sitting in a conference room brainstorming session, came up with the term one day to soften it up.

The person at the window set up my CT-Scan, blood draw (which this place called Labs) and my next Doctors appointment. I asked about my next chemo. It would be four weeks, on my next doctor's appointment.

"Oh don't worry, the doctor will decide what you need, and we will get you in on time, the latest it would be is Tuesday, only one day late."

"You're sure?" I wasn't taking any chances.

"Let us worry. You just work on getting healthy."

I left feeling a little confused by all of it, but better about my doctors and the team that worked with him than I did at the other place. Of course, I felt good about them at first too. At least, this place had people walk you to where you need to be, and the doctor actually talked to you about your chemotherapy and what he was doing rather than saying, "It's protocol."

CHAPTER TWENTY-EIGHT
FOOLING YOURSELF

I went for my CT-Scan at a hospital connected to this cancer center. I can't tell you how much better I felt right from the time I entered the room. It was a little complicated getting to the correct place as we were sent from room to room to check in. However once I entered the actual suite where the scan took place, I was greeted promptly; there wasn't an over- crowding/overbooking issue, and I didn't have to refill out paperwork! Once I was entered into the computer on the first day, which took care of the repetitive questions that every department seemed to ask in the former hospital.

It only took a few minutes for a nurse to call my name. She took me back to a private room, and started the IV that the contrast IV would eventually be hooked into. It was nice when I explained to her that a butterfly worked best on me and that I only had one good vein for a thicker needle and what happened when the girls didn't use that spot.

She tapped the one vein I pointed out, and said, *"Wow, if that's the juiciest vein you have you really do need a butterfly!"* I liked her sense of humor and the fact that she listened to me. She handed me my drink which was cold for a change, and she asked if I wanted some strawberry-kiwi flavor added. I said sure I'd try it. The flavoring was nice, but making it cold was great for me. I always drank all my beverages with a lot of ice. So with my usual flair, I pounded the drink and took the cup back.

"Wow! You have done this before! Ok I've noted the time. Someone will come get you in just under an hour." She told me where the rest room was if I needed it, clarifying that it wasn't necessary for me to hold my urine. How very nice, instructions right from the start!

Forty minutes later a tall gentleman in a white coat came up to me, identified himself and asked me to repeat my name and birthdate then instructed me to follow him. He walked me back to a room with the same machine as the last hospital. He asked if I tolerated the contrast well. I said no, and then he was very specific.

"Does it bother you right when it starts or when you feel it reaching your head?"

I remembered the last time when I had felt like it was creeping up on my head and I could taste it. Then that overwhelming feeling of nausea.

"When it gets to my head."

"Ok, I can work with that."

He gave me a blanket and had me lay on the table. Again moving my pants down to my knees, he hooked his part of the IV up. Within seconds the machine was running and the table I lay on was moving. He took many more pictures than the last hospital, and as I could feel the chemicals reaching my mouth I heard his voice:

"Kim, can you taste it?"

"Yes."

Again, without pause, I heard him rush into the room and disconnect the IV contrast.

"Just a couple more pictures real quick. Hold on just a few more seconds, did the taste stop?"

"Yes."

"Are you feeling ok?"

"Yes."

And with that, again hurried footsteps and the machine and pictures started again. With only a few minutes having passed, he was back by my side.

"Ok, I'm going to take the rest of this IV out now and you can get up slowly and take your time to get settled. I will wait behind the door. He removed the IV, and I heard the door slam behind him. I sat up slowly. I felt much better than the last two times, and I tried to think, he must have taken six maybe eight pictures. I looked at my phone. I had been in the room less than fifteen minutes, and I didn't feel like vomiting. He re-entered the room after asking if I was all set, and escorted me back to the main waiting room. He also said what my nurse had said.

"Page your nurse on Thursday if you want to know your results or you can wait for your next doctor's appointment. It's totally up to you."

With that, I was done. No crowded rooms, no sick people coughing on me, no extended stay, and no sickness. That made me feel better.

✦ ✦

On Thursday at 1pm, I took out my card and paged the nurse. I tried to time it where it wasn't too early in the morning or lunchtime, and there was enough hours left in the work day to call back. Twenty minutes later my phone rang.

"Hi, this is So-and-So, somebody paged me?"

"Hi, it's Kim Henderly. I was calling about the results of my CT-Scan?"

"Oh sure. Hi Kim. Let me pull those up right now."

I was impressed. Whether she really knew who I was really was irrelevant. She made me feel like she did, and she called from a place and at a time where she could answer my question immediately; not give me a song and dance about having to look it up and call me back.

Unfortunately, the news wasn't as good as I had hoped. Just as I had thought, there was cancer present in a few spots, plus the higher up areas that I had asked to be scanned (and they never did) showed a 4mm nodule.

I wanted nothing more than to hang up and call a lawyer and sue the former hospital and every person I had had contact with. Two weeks before, their idiot radiologist read my scan as clear. Obviously this new doctor didn't see those scans the same way, and thankfully, had ordered these additional scans like I asked.

I told The Other and my sisters, that if I die in these upcoming rounds of chemotherapy because they couldn't get back in front of this disease, that I wanted them all to sue the hospital. I resigned myself to more chemo but kept the same outlook. I will do this and be done, then be in another remission.

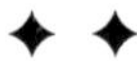

I saw the doctor a second time on the following Monday.

This cancer center had its own way of handling chemotherapy. I showed up at 9 am and went to the lab/infusion center. I checked in by name and birthday and about ten minutes later a nurse called my name. They escort you back to one of two rooms. One if you took your chemo through a vein, the other room for people with ports like mine. I had to have my port x-rayed on my first doctor's visit here, since this center didn't install it, they wanted 'a picture' on record. The room had a half dozen chairs and a nurse for each chair. They took vitals, asked specific questions as to exactly how I was feeling, such as pain level, any sickness, and bathroom regularity as well as questions about my emotions, depression and the need for a social worker for assistance. Then the nurse inserted the end of the IV into the port, drew blood, and sent the vials to the lab in a dumbwaiter right in front of me.

From there, it was back to the clinic to check in with the doctor. He more thoroughly explained what was on the CT scans and his opinion on how to proceed with chemotherapy that day. They were going to keep the Taxol/Carbo for three rounds and do another CT-Scan. If there was no improvement, they would change my meds. Even with the big file from the previous hospital, I felt like they didn't have enough information to go on, but I liked the fact that he wanted another scan right away. No playing around. The doctor talked to me for about a half an hour on how he treats different patients with ovarian cancer, their reactions, and his thoughts. He listened carefully when I asked questions and gave me full answers once again. He also asked if there was anything I had read or heard about, and if I didn't understand it, to ask someone and once again pointed out his nurse as a wealth of information.

Then he was very specific about him being my doctor. Not the nurses who administer chemotherapy or anyone else in the hospital. Questions were to go to him, and if anyone didn't treat me well or called into question anything, I was to let him know. I liked that. I felt like he was in charge of my care and used a support staff correctly.

From the clinic, it was back to the Lab/Infusion Center, where you check in and wait. This varied as the months went on from forty-five minutes to ninety minutes. Essentially, you checked back in, and they ordered your meds from the pharmacy. Once those meds arrived, I was called back to a private room with a hospital bed, two chairs, TV, sink, and a small nurse's stand. It was quiet, private, and comfortable.

My first infusion nurse at this facility was a very pretty woman about my age. She was fun and talkative, and an incredible wealth of knowledge to get me through my first treatment at the facility. She listened to my whole story, shared her story, and gave me information on things that might help me with side-effects from the medicines. I liked her a lot. I liked the chemotherapy nurse at the other hospital, but I felt like this woman really had it going on when it came to knowledge, and she didn't have to backhand feed me information in order to 'follow some rule.' She was never out of line and didn't contradict the doctor like the nurses at the other hospital did. She spent a great deal of time with me on that first treatment. I didn't feel like I was rushed or that she was rushed. I was very grateful.

By the time I got through labs, the doctor's visit and chemotherapy, I had been at the hospital for more than eight hours. It was too long of a day for me, but I actually felt really great compared to the previous chemotherapy treatments. I did feel bad for my mother-in-law. She was the one driving me and having to sit there all day and wait while I went through all these steps. It was hard on me; I knew it had to be even worse for her.

The last hospital at lunch brought out a cold sandwich, cookie and a half can of pop. For lunch here, there was soup and a sandwich, yogurt, fruit and juice or water. It was a large healthy lunch served by wonderful senior volunteers. The extra large portions were great and helped with a later day snack. They also offered Sue coffee and water throughout the day. An aide stopped by to get vitals during treatment a few times. At the last place, they hooked you up to a blood pressure cuff and left it on your arm.

Before I left for the day, they gave me a copy of all my labs and numbers without having to ask and a calendar with my next appointment only three short weeks away.

Most importantly, I went to work the next day and felt okay. Was

I a hundred percent? No, but I hadn't been that good since remission. The fact that I could get up, get dressed, and go to work without feeling like I was going to heave every two seconds was good with me.

I wish I could say that good feeling lasted. I worked from home the rest of the week and part of the second week. The side-effects on this round were not only the usual barrage of hard-hitting gastric distress issues that kept me glued to the toilet but they were also encompassing my mouth. My tongue felt like the entire length of it had a hot-cheese-pizza-slice scald the surface, even the sides of my tongue felt burnt. My throat was the same deteriorating situation as if I was having a case of strep for more than a week without the aid of medication. The porcelain crown that I had had put in years ago was suffering as the gums in that area started to recede; every bite of food was painful and forced me to remove the particles of food that had become lodged in the gum area around the crown.

Now stop for a minute. Put the book down and make yourself something soft to eat, like a sandwich on soft bread. Take one small bite and chew, and then floss your teeth. Take another small soft bite and floss again, over and over; try to consume an entire sandwich by the bite-and-floss method. This tedious task became mine for five days! I even stopped chewing on the one side, another daunting task; only, that process aggravated the other side of the tongue even more!

Having this new side-effect, as well as the itchy-head that comes with the brand-new hair fallout and the inability to have a decent bowel moment without digging it out by hand, proved that I was at a tipping point. The hair caught me by surprise. It had been eight months between the treatments, and my hair was even shorter than the last time it had fallen out, but it had grown back thick, like it was in my twenties, so I chalked the itchiness up to more hair taking longer to fall out. Over three treatments to be exact. The itchiness was driving me crazy!

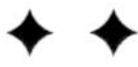

When I was at the cancer center for treatment, I was shown a library with a ton of information on any type of cancer you could think of. I grabbed everything I could find relating to ovarian cancer, cancer's return and healthy lifestyles. I started to read again; the booklets were a re-hash of everything I had been reading on line, and the healthy lifestyles turned out to be the government recommendations of a 'balanced' diet. I was still not getting the information I felt I needed.

I couldn't possibly be the only person in the world suffering this much. So it was back to the computer. This time I started to type into Google:

Ovarian cancer returns.

Here is where knowing the correct terminology comes in to play when doing research… and after months of typing things like 'Ovarian Cancer' 'Ovarian Cancer Side Effects' I started to type 'ovarian cancer returns' and got as far as–Ovarian Cancer RE, and the word RECURRENT popped up. That led me to a new site: "Cancerconnect.com." It was here that I first learned about the difference between persistent, refractory or recurrent cancer. It was also here that I knew every hope that every person had given me was ripped away.

The worst and most emotionally draining of the three was recurrent. Given the fact that most ovarian cancer patients had a twelve to eighteen months chance of survival after the first reoccurrence with fewer than one in ten making it to five years, the other two teetered in that two to five year span. I was devastated. I felt like once again I had been lied to and I didn't understand the methodology behind it. Why when I woke up from the surgery, over a year ago now, when I asked the question about *"what are my chances?"* was I not told… *"You are terminal"* …I know doctors aren't fortune tellers. They cannot replace God. Nobody can 'predict' death, but I would have liked to have known from the start that there was less than a 50/50 chance that I wouldn't make it to five years and then let me develop my own hope and drive. Instead, I was fed such a line of shit! With these three new words *persistent, refractory and recurrent,* I added them to the words *ovarian cancer* and the real numbers started to come up. The numbers were flying at my chances of making it on this reoccurrence at less than two years, and they got really low for five years and were almost nonexistent for ten.

I knew cancer wasn't a winning game with anyone. But I went

into this at first believing they could rid me of it. If I was one of the lucky few, I thought, at least, I had about ten years left. Now I starting to look at the picture differently, and I needed to plan differently. There was a strong chance that as I sat there three months into my second go round with the same cancer in under a year's time that I wasn't going to make it to see my fiftieth birthday.

I sat in a chair, shades drawn staring at my living room. The house packing was well on its way. The boxes along the living room wall were neatly stacked floor to ceiling and labeled. The shelves were empty, and I could see the autumn sun through the window blinds that covered our extra-large window. What have I done to myself? How the hell did this happen? I had involved myself in a child's life and now I was going to drop out of site forever. I thought about all the pain I was going to inflict on people by dying. My mom! They say there is no greater pain than losing a child. My dad was getting sicker every single day, and soon she would lose a man she had been with for almost fifty-five years and then her oldest child. I didn't want to be that person, yet I didn't know what to do to prevent it from happening. I was at a loss for the first time in my life as to what to do with myself, and I knew I had to tell my close friends and family what was going on. I sat down and composed an email to my sisters and parents and wrote an open letter to my close friends on a social media site. I laid it all out there and what my 'real' chances of survival were. I cried as I wrote the letter and the email and asked that nobody contact me until I got my head around the idea of my own, now certain, untimely death.

Then, I crawled into bed for two days and cried, while the chemo ravaged my body for another month.

Hidden in the clouds above
You can feel them looking down
They are hard to see, but it's easy to believe
There are angels all around

- Kim Henderly

CHAPTER TWENTY-NINE

ANDREA AND KAREN: THE ANGELS AMONG US

Cancer is like any medical problem in this country; in which we have some of the best tests in the world. However there is always a wait to get results. The waiting is always the hardest. You have to hurry up, get tested, and wait days for the results. Nobody calls you as soon as they arrive—you have to wait the appropriate amount of time, and by that I mean a few days, sometimes up to a week. You can't call for results too soon because then you are greeted with the dreaded 'someone will call you back.' That could take up to a week in itself, for a nurse to sit down at a desk and make all her calls (you're dreaming if you think the doctor is going to call you personally). If you are lucky and time it right, you will get to talk to a nurse or some girl working the front desk. Usually, a soft, calm, professional voice who can tell you the results and nothing else, except come in and the doctor will talk to you about what those results mean to you. You get to wait again in an even more precarious position of 'a little knowledge.' One of two things will happen as you wait for an appointment with a small amount of knowledge: you either get a 'not you,' and I will be totally ok, or you get the worst case scenario vibe–fueled by bad, too general internet information or days of an upset stomach diarrhea and lack of appetite. Well-meaning friends and family will want to do things with you to keep your mind occupied (ask them to pay and by all means go!) The more you keep your mind and body active the better off you are. Middle ground is illusive and hard to control. I found myself wavering between all these things. Upset and thinking the worst one minute and completely convinced that I was the lucky one and all the tests were wrong the next.

When the follow up appointment finally comes, you arrive, and you wait again. My average wait time was over ninety minutes to actually talk to the doctor–in most cases, I wanted to move to the next step to know the actual specific results of the test and go to the next treatment. Everything is an emergency and time-sensitive when it comes to cancer, and people were being 'fit in' all the time. Every time I sat in a waiting room, I saw the newly-diagnosed. I wondered if I looked like that when I started the process. One woman in particular caught my eye while I was waiting at the clinic. She was well-dressed, expensive leather coat, hair recently dyed and styled, her husband's loafers polished to a brilliant shine. Her daughter looked to be in her early twenties, long blonde hair and her nose in her phone. She never said a word to her mom. Just looked around the room at the other patients in disgust. I couldn't help but think that this girl has a long way to go to develop a bit of compassion that is going to be needed to be able to come here and sit with her mom. Dad kept getting up, picking literature up off the table and reading it to his wife. She sat there like a deer in headlights, staring at the people as they came and went. In my first rounds of chemotherapy, over a year ago now, I looked like the sickest person in the room. The surgery had made me that way. Here at this cancer center, I looked like one of the healthier patients. I wanted to walk across the waiting room and talk to her, tell her the truth and what to ask the doctor when she went in. I knew by looking at her that what the doctor was about to tell her was going to be lost. She was checked out, upset, and out of her element in this cancer center.

I had been on one of my 'waiting for test results' weeks, and it was starting to get to me and then I saw a social media status post about my friend Andrea. She was slipping, and her husband had a scare a few nights earlier and almost lost her. It wasn't but a few days after that that I received a text telling me of her passing.

Andrea was a woman a few years younger than me. Our paths had crossed several times through the joy and merriment of music and friends. We had always smiled at each other; I remember how beautiful she had always looked so put-together, so friendly, so full of life as if nothing could break her happiness. Who would have thought that something so incredibly ugly, hurtful, and ridiculously untreatable such as cancer would bond us together.

Ten months earlier, her husband had put a status update about seizures and an unknown illness, which turned out, after much testing, to be a brain tumor. She went through surgery and radiation, as well as Avastin. She accepted it all and never once complained about how hard it all was. I contacted her husband an offered up any support or information he needed while she was in the hospital. Andrea contacted me right after her hospital stay and the four of us met for dinner to talk.

She called me her hero for fighting so hard, going on with my life, job, relationships and laughing in the face of cancer. I envied her for being able to dismiss every negative thing the doctors told her and push forward in an unstoppable way.

We talked privately about treatments as the months went on, IM'd and emailed when we could. She had her support group and circle of friends that I didn't want to intrude on with my own cancer issues, but a day didn't go by that I didn't think about her or talk to her in my own way when I was feeling like shit from side effects.

Andrea was never going to give up. She tried everything and traveled everywhere to send herself into remission, and now she was again back in the hospital and fading fast. It scared the hell out of me. I knew I was nowhere near as positive of survival at this point as she had been, yet she was losing her battle quickly, too quickly. If she couldn't beat this, I sure in the hell couldn't.

The day I got the text about her losing the fight, I was floundering on the couch five day's into my own horrible side-effects. The problems were so strong and unrelenting during this round that I was desperately trying to figure out how I was going to make it through another month. I didn't think I had it in me to move forward. On the couch, I lie, praying for God to somehow grant me more strength so I could stick around and finish help with the move to the new house and take care of Chris and Hunter for a little longer when the phone beeped. Jenn Balcom had been on the other end of her phone debating whether or not she should tell me or wait until I was feeling better. The news hit me hard. I have been sad before when someone had passed away, but this was an incredible hurt. I was so upset. Andrea had pushed so hard, was so positive about her life. I felt I didn't have half the strength she had. I cried for hours, alone on the couch. I cried because I knew one day it will be me that people are gathering by the bedside for, hoping for a peaceful end, and praying for a miracle. I cried because I knew the pain in My Other's eye's every time we got more bad news, and I have seen that same look in her husband's eyes. Teri tells me, she gets mad, throws things, destroys what reminds her of her survival and someone else's limited time. I don't feel that anger. I feel the pain. The pain for those who are left without their friend, their sister, their confident, his soul mate; she is somebody's daughter, a person who makes you happy that you know her.

I have nothing to offer but my written word. I wish that was enough to wipe away the pain, the hurt, the loss of energy that anyone who knew her will now feel. I don't pretend to be anything more than what I am: someone who was lucky enough, if only for a brief moment to have called her my friend. She is my hero too, for never ever giving up and fighting until the bitter end.

This stupid disease has created another Angel way before her time.

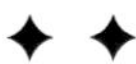

Immediately following Andrea, came, Karen, a woman I had worked with for many years.

Over time, Karen, a third friend, Michelle, and I had become close. Every day for more than a decade going into the same job. A job that encompassed the 1990's and well into the recession of the mid 2000's. The work place, for the three of us, was more like a therapy session in life some mornings. As we all attended our daily tasks, we talked through problems and discussions began. We all gave our opinions and then the person in crisis for the moment could make a calculated choice on what was bothering them. Karen helped me through some of the worst issues in my life at the time. She was grounded and wise.

She had contracted Hodgkin's Lymphoma about the same time I was diagnosed. She was also my age. Karen fought on for a while. She had to give up her job in order to be able to go on public assistance to get treatment. Now here was someone who worked her entire life yet she had no health insurance, because health insurance isn't offered in her line of work—the hospitality industry. I could only think... that could have been me had I not be introduced to my current company owners.

She fought and dealt with the side-effects. Until she couldn't anymore. You see chemotherapy is a monster. However life is not a video game. There were no swords, special weapons that glow or even a programming cheat. It's a monster that you have to take on yourself. And no matter who stands with you, you are still fighting alone. She lost her internal need to fight. Karen made peace with herself and let the chips fall where they may. She stopped her chemotherapy. She left us a month after Andrea, leaving behind two children and a family that loved her dearly. Chemotherapy and cancer had won and beaten her down.

I couldn't help to think after Andrea and Karen's untimely deaths that something was terribly wrong in this country. Cancer had become a major money-making machine and even with the best-laid intentions of the tens of thousands of volunteers and inspirational survivors, we really had only added a few years, and in some cases only a few months to life and mildly improved side-effects of the treatment of this deadly killer. We had better screening on *some* cancers and nothing for others. The squeaky wheel got the grease in this country. Some very wealthy women along with their family and friends put breast cancer on the map, and Katie Couric, who I am guessing, watched her husband suffer a great deal, also tried to make a big statement and get people's attention. It takes an experience like mine with side-effects from treatment, and the gut-wrenching terror of losing your life's love to go on a number-one rated national television show and have a colonoscopy, but she did for that cancer and its victims. She did what needed to be done. She set aside the jokes I am sure she knew would follow, the embarrassment of what the procedure actually does, and she sucked it up and showed people that anyone could have the procedure done, and it could save you so much physical pain and heartache. She took what I am sure was a generation of people saying, "You're not sticking that thing up my ass" to a point where they thought twice about it and at least asked a doctor or listened when a doctor talked about it.... Go back and reread my chapter on side-effects. I am telling you she is correct. Being put under anesthesia and checked is by far the better choice between the two.

Yes, we were making strides. However, they were not enough. I started to think about all the beds and chairs, not just in this new cancer hospital but in the place that I had been treated in previously. I knew that within an hour's drive from my own house there were also six more centers that I could think of. To me, that meant thousands of people every day filling those chairs—poison dripping slowly through their veins, fighting to remain here with their friends and family; it also meant money. Millions of dollars every day pouring out; cancer employed a lot of people in a very bad economy, and it kept the coffers very full indeed. Stories were starting to come out about how cancer medications were becoming scarcer with the price rising far faster than it should, no insurance? No problem! The government would step in and pay via government-assisted medical programs. Someone was getting very wealthy on the backs of many dying people. The cost of my treatment was rising, and the drugs I was going to need as this went forward were becoming more and more unavailable. Black market chemotherapy drugs were popping up everywhere, and some were found to be not the actual drug but a watered-down substitute. This is some consolation that the government is "looking into it" when a four-year-old's mother has been killed because she was given a 'fake' chemotherapy drug, so some douchebag can sit and drink twenty-five-year-old scotch on his yacht surrounded by gold-digging groupies.

These thoughts are all political hot button issues, which people can get very riled up about. In the eyes of a person dying from cancer, they are an emotional rollercoaster on the road to never-ending hopelessness.

The only thing you want is to survive. The only thing you are handed is excuses as to why you can't. You watch every news show that promises new information on cancer, only to find out that the latest breakthroughs' are usually still way out of your lifespan to do you any good.

It is about this time in your treatment, when you have a full knowledge of what is really going to happen to you. You can get your head around how hard the treatment will continue to be, and that you will be broke from the medical bills. Then you have to make your true choice....

Give up or fight.

I had seen both sides now; Andrea had never let the word terminal into her vocabulary and fought until the moment she took her last breath. Karen had chosen to end her painful treatments and let nature take its course.

I knew what people thought of me. I heard it daily. Quite frankly I needed to hear it daily.

"You are the strongest person I know. If anyone can beat this you can."

I hated that phrase. I never felt strong when I was vomiting uncontrollably, or wriggling in pain as my legs were out of control. I only felt helpless and alone. Like no one really understood what I was going through on a monthly basis. What did it really mean to be strong? That I was able to 'tolerate' the embarrassment of having to dig my own shit out of my ass? Or that I was capable of holding my head high while walking around the mall without eyebrows, eyelashes and hair ignoring the stares? I never felt 'strong.' As I mourned both their deaths, I also talked to and watched the pain it caused to the people they loved. The fear I had most was not my own mortality. I personally have a very strong belief in Heaven and what is waiting for us beyond this realm. However, I didn't want my family and friends to suffer the emotional pain that I knew would come and was confirmed in watching the passing of these two women. As this power was taking over me, I received a phone call while waiting to see my oncologist for my next treatment. It was from our third coworker, Michelle, from the days when we all worked together.

I had been thinking about the new patient, her husband and disconnected daughter in the waiting room and speaking to her when my phone started vibrating...

I heard Michelle's voice on the other end of the phone begin to talk about Karen. Michelle never said I was strong; she called me and asked me *"to never give up, never quit fighting."* She was also upset by Karen's passing and didn't understand her decision to give up. She begged me to keep on going and not to walk away from treatment. Over and over, the same words came out of her mouth. I took that as the same challenge Chris would give me every month as I suffered through side-effects. I remembered Hunter's words about not leaving him here.

Andrea and Karen's death gave me something. It wasn't that I needed to be strong; it was that I needed another reason to fight; I needed to know that someone, anyone still wanted me here. Michelle, Karen, and I were very tight for a long time, and our lives had taken us to explore different parts of this very large world we all live in. Yet, she still held on to those memories of the three of us, and she wasn't ready to let go, to let me go. All along I had been looking for a reason to stop the side-effects, to stop the pain. I wasn't strong at all, but I was always up for a good challenge, a dare, or a bet that I couldn't accomplish something, and as the fog of the reality of my now fully-realized terminal status set in, it was a matter of feeling sorry for myself or playing the odds.

Chris needed me. Hunter needed me. My sisters and parents needed me, and the first of my friends had actually come out and said, *"I will kick your ass if you give up."*

My goal, to be part of the less than twenty percent to make it to ten years; I was comfortable with that number and I was one year into that goal. First, there was the hard part...

I turned to smile at the lady's husband as he approached the table next to my chair to look for something else to read about cancer. He reminded me of me in the beginning, trying to read my way through it. He smiled back and commented:

"There sure is a lot of information lying around here."

I was quick to respond *"And the library over there is full of booklets. Don't forget to stop in there: too bad all this information doesn't tell you what you really need to know about your wife's ovarian cancer."*

"How did you know she had ovarian cancer?"

"You are sitting in the Ovarian Clinic." I guess he didn't listen to his tour guide on the way in either.

"Oh, yeah right." He smiled awkwardly. *"Listen, do you mind if I ask you a few questions?"*

I agreed and talked to him and then his wife and daughter for the next thirty minutes until they called my name. When I emerged from the exam room the three of them were still sitting there. I paused to say goodbye when the woman said:

"We've been waiting here a long time."

I smiled. *"Get used to it. You will spend the rest of your time waiting for everything—from doctor's visits to test results. They will tell you don't stress. I say find something to do to keep yourself busy. You'll find your own niche."*

They thanked me, and I was on my way. I have run into the lady and her daughter several times since then. We always talk for a few minutes and over the course of these conversations, I found her story to have traits similar to mine, from the misdiagnosis to the lack of information on side-effects. She thanked me for being honest about the side-effects and said I was the only one who was that she's met so far. I watched as her beautiful hair was replaced by a wig and the expensive clothes by sweat pants and pajamas. The makeup was gone and her daughter held her hand and talked to her, barely looking at her phone. The process had aged her. Where when I first saw her in the waiting room that day, I would have thought she was a well put together fifty something easily pulling off looking like she was in her late forties. Now, she looked older than the sixty-one years that she had told me she was.

CHAPTER THIRTY
MOVING

Three short weeks after my first chemotherapy infusion at this new cancer hospital, I was back in the private room, sitting on the bed with the IV drip going. It was Halloween of 2011, and for the second year in a row, I had missed one of the fun holidays I usually spent with friends.

I had grown accustomed to the fiscal austerity imposed on me by overwhelming medical bills, but I was still having an issue, off and on, with the not being able to go out in large crowds and party like I used to.

The doctors and other professionals in the field don't insist, but strongly suggest that you stay out of large crowds especially during cold and flu season and when your numbers are all on the low side. My numbers were their lowest during third week, which meant on a three week rotation of chemo instead of the usual four, I was sick for two weeks and unable to go anywhere. Then, there was my quarantine week and back to chemo. I wanted to get into another remission as soon as possible. However, this new routine wasn't making me happy as a whole person, and I wasn't quite sold on it. I was to put it bluntly… Housebound.

I asked for my numbers as soon as I hit the bed. I wanted to know if three weeks was going to make a big difference. I was happy when I saw the CA125 post in the low 500's. Yet, I couldn't help but think that I wouldn't be sitting here with my fourth round of chemo starting, and I was not at the CA125 -100 mark where I was in the last round by treatment four. It told me that the numbers that they kept from me had shot way up over the 1640 I had been told at the other cancer center. It also confirmed that I had done the correct thing by switching doctors and facilities. Yet, I wasn't stupid and not being platinum sensitive meant the chemo was working. That was a good thing, but I would need a minimum of six more rounds of this stuff. The nurse that was administering the infusion pointed out my white counts. They were on the lowest side of normal possible. She was going to call and let the doctor know because I was going to need a shot of Neulasta. Neulasta was the latest and greatest at raising a person's white counts. It was expensive, but it worked 100% of the time. She explained that I would have to come back to the cancer hospital twenty-four hours after chemo had concluded and they would give me a shot of the medicine, and it would help raise my white counts. I agreed and signed all the paper work. When chemo finished, they told me to arrive the next day sometime after 4 pm but before they closed at 7 pm.

I finished up that infusion round and headed home to start with the horrific side-effects that I knew were coming. Although this new place seemed to really have it together and have my best interests at heart, the side-effects hadn't mellowed at all. I had actually added to them. I had met with the doctor three times already, the resident in a one-on-one fashion twice, and the oncology nurse. I had been very specific about the constipation and vomiting, which in my mind were the ones that I was having issues dealings with. They were all patient and offered up the best advice they had, and I had followed every instruction to the letter, yet I was getting no relief. I had resolved myself to prayer in hopes that God would give me the strength to tolerate it as best as I could.

On November 1st, my part-time status started back at work, and in eleven days, we were closing on the new house. I was hoping that the distraction of finishing getting the house ready would help me. For the next week, I would sit on a chair and pack one box and then lay down to rest. During the periods of insomnia, I would do my office work. Having work to do passed the time for me in the early morning hours and made the nights seem shorter. On that day, I also had to drive myself in rush hour back downtown to the hospital. I hated making this ride and so wished they would open a treatment center near my home. I showed up, checked in at the lab, and within five minutes was back in the nurses' chair with them asking the same questions they do before chemotherapy and taking my vitals. The Neulasta arrived from the pharmacy, and I had a choice of a shot in the back of my upper arm or in the stomach. I choose the upper arm, and after a quick pick and a small burning sensation when the medicine was shot in my arm, there was really nothing to it. I asked about side-effects and was told that nobody really has any that any of the nurses working in the room had heard of, but they printed me an official sheet of side-effects. Knowing how prone I was to side-effects on this whole process, I wanted to know everything. When I got home I laughed, when reading the sheet 'nausea,' 'constipation,' and 'diarrhea' caught my eye. Really? Do these pharmaceutical companies print the same list out for every drug? Once again, how do you have 'constipation' and 'diarrhea' at the same time? It made no difference. I was headed for side-effect hell again and figured the effects from that drug would blend in with the rest.

I was wrong–again. I went through my side-effects as usual feeling a little better by the following Monday. Week two after chemo had always been an unknown for me. I would struggle wanting desperately to come out of side-effects, but things would linger. Each day, I would get a little better. By the weekend, I could usually move about freely. This time was the same except that a full ten days after treatment, after I thought I was 'out of the woods' so to speak, I got the chills. It was winter in Michigan. I turned up the heat in the house, put on my robe over my sweater and jeans, and tried to pack more. I left to pick up Hunter and came home and couldn't get warm. I asked The Little One if he was cold.

"No. It's way hotter than usual in here," came his response.

I changed into pajamas, put my robe back on and crawled under the covers in bed. I called for Hunter to bring me another blanket from the living room, and he volunteered to make me soup. I ate the soup and laid watching TV under the blankets; by the time Chris got home, I was in full blown shiver. He tried to warm me up, and it wasn't long after that I was rushing into the bathroom, vomit and diarrhea exploding from my body.

"WHAT THE HELL IS GOING ON NOW!!!!" I screamed.

I was angry. Why was I going through another round of this!?! I wanted to punch the wall. Eight days of torture wasn't enough. Now I was sick again. Two additional times, I got sick that night. Afterwards, I nibbled saltines and sipped ginger ale. The chills stopped as soon as I got sick. I went and lay on the couch and opened up my laptop. I googled "Neulasta problems" and found a thread from a forum that was based in Germany. I learned a lot that night. Reading post after post, Neulasta takes about ten days to kick in and that chills, vomiting and diarrhea follow but then it's over. People were suggesting all types of weird things to combat the side-effects. I read them knowing I wouldn't do any of them since all my efforts to ward off side-effects were useless with chemo, and this was all part of it. I knew that nothing was going to help me. I went on the company site for the drug and read about it. I wasn't pleased at all when I learned that one of the issues with the drug is that it "could make cancer cells grow". ***How stupid was this? You give me a drug to help with low white counts because of cancer treatment only to have the treatment make the cancer reproduce itself?*** I saw a money pattern forming in that statement.

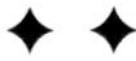

It was coming up on our closing date. I had been vomiting on the 9th and the 10th of November. The day before closing required a walkthrough of the house we were buying. My real estate agent knew about my cancer, but I let no one else that was involved with the house know. I was afraid they would hold it against me. As the closing date arrived, I woke that morning and donned my wig and full makeup to head out with The Other to closing. I managed to drive myself to the walk-through the day before, and all of the mortgage information was done via phone and internet so I never had to physically see anyone from the mortgage company.

I am sure that on the day of closing the lady from the Title Company, the seller's agent and the seller had no idea at all that I was sick in any way. That really is sad. I thought about the thousands of people daily who hide their illness from friends, coworkers, and the general public wanting not to be judged. The feeling was humiliating. It gave me a new respect for people who had to deal with being judged on a daily basis.

At the end of my last rounds of treatment and all through this treatment, I made it known fully to everyone I had cancer. Then, shortly thereafter, I focused on the fact that the cancer was terminal. I felt it was necessary that everyone knew I was suffering with this disease, and I didn't want to hide anything from the world. The fact that I had to hide for fear of repercussion–such as not getting a loan, which I was more than qualified for, irritated me.

My own real estate agent had become more than a business associate over the years of working with and for her. We had developed a conversational friendship, and I felt she needed to know the truth about my cancer. As we did the walk thru the day before closing, the two of us in the basement of what was to be our new abode I told her. Her tears spoke volumes. Many of my friends are like me and try to hold back these emotions for my sake. She was visibly shaken, and she gave me a hug. I remember telling her:

"Don't worry; I've come to terms with it."

Knowing full well that saying those words and actually doing it were two different things, but I knew she would feel better if I said that.

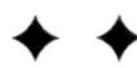

Three weeks later, on November 21, I showed up at the cancer hospital, had my labs drawn and sat down for a fourth time to talk to the doctor. I was not afraid of starting another chemo infusion in three short weeks, but I was worried about my quality of life.

Again, a new side-effect had started in this past round. The bottom of my left foot was numb and so were the tips of my thumb and index finger on both hands. This combined with the added illness of the drug to pump up my white cells was taking its toll on me. I read up on the 'numbness' that was listed on all the cancer websites, and like the mouth issues from last month, this month added another problem. I wondered why on the last go-round of six treatments I had not experienced this. I was headed into treatment number five and still under the amount of infusions as last time to be having these two new issues.

I found a site that helped explain the numbness, which was actually called neuropathy. It is a common side-effect. When I first read about numbness in the hands and feet, I thought about my carpal tunnel. I assumed I could handle it because I was used to that pins-and-needles kind of feeling. Unfortunately, and unlike carpal tunnel where you can shake your hands around and get some blood moving through your hands to relieve the feeling, you can't do that with numbness caused by neuropathy. It comes and stays with you. It also increases with every treatment in severity and the span of the body that it covers.

When you put those two new side-effects up, with the fact that I only was now getting about nine good days where I could function in what I would consider a 'livable' fashion (if you consider livable to mean you can't go into a crowd), I wasn't really sold on the whole three weeks thing. I knew it was the preferred protocol at this cancer center but was it the best treatment for me. This new schedule was taking away my quality of life. A life that was very limited.

Before the doctor walked in my exam room, a new resident came in and sat down. I thought I would try again and told her all about the side-effects, in addition to the new ones. She offered up nothing new. She went through a dozen 'fixes,' and I told her I had tried all of them as she listed them. She conceded in the end that it's all part of the side-effects of the medicine and that I probably couldn't do anything else.

As the doctor arrived, with my file in hand and sat down, I told him of my concern about the two new side effects and the fact that I didn't like only having a week of normal living.

My doctor had always commented when he came in the room about 'how good I looked.' I know what he meant; not that I was some hottie sitting there, but that I was walking under my own power, sitting upright, not incessantly complaining. I was well-dressed and usually had a bit of color in my skin. I saw many of his patients in wheelchairs, all of whom looked extremely ill. I was not one of those. Actually, unless you came to my house during a side-effect week, you probably wouldn't know I was ill, especially if I was in full makeup and wig. I used the fact that my doctor saw that in me to plead my case.

"I look good and feel better I think because I have a couple weeks to get my strength back. If you want me to tolerate all this chemo, you have to give me a chance to recoup. I don't think I can do this every three weeks. So unless you tell me it's detrimental to my life, I want to do four weeks."

He agreed, and I was relieved. If my days here on earth were numbered, I wanted to at least be able to function. Not be reduced to a mess lying in bed every day and to being wheeled in for treatments; that seemed ludicrous to me.

The doctor took the opportunity that I was going to be back on four weeks to ask me if I wanted to also try Avastin. He wanted me to but was leaving the final decision up to me.

Avastin had been in the news in the past few days. The FDA had recalled its use because they felt it did not add enough significant time to a breast cancer patient's life. That meant for me to use it, my insurance company would have to approve its use in my particular case with my particular cancer.

First, let me explain. Avastin and its generic counterparts work by preventing tumors from forming the little veins they do and connecting with a person's blood supply which then feeds the tumor and helps it grow. Thus the tumor loses its food source, shrivels up, and dies. To use this medicine you would have to have a tumor-based cancer.

For those who like to take an all-natural and healthy approach to life, you can find many studies on green tea, which when consumed in large quantities (more than thirty-two ounces a day for most people) and on a daily basis (without fail), green tea is said to lend itself to the same effect. I had been told about green tea from a nutritionist and a dietician and had read many reports and studies on it. I had also been consuming exactly thirty-two ounces a day for about eight months at the point I was asked about the Avastin.

The doctor asked if I knew what Avastin was and what it did, and not waiting for an answer explained exactly what it did. He gave his opinion on the FDA and their findings and then let me decide. I thought, why not, I was already on a whole host of medications, what was one more.

"If you think it might help, and you are moving me to four weeks, let's

do it. But tell me the worst side-effects because I have had a bad track record with side-effects, and I will probably get whatever is listed."

He thought that the worst case scenario was a nose bleed and to let him know if that happened.

The nurse disconnected the IV that was started for my infusion, and I was sent home with instructions to return in one week. I was elated that they started by moving my treatment to the four weeks. I had done three weeks twice, and I didn't think I could handle it again. I also knew that I had scheduled movers for the next day, and Thanksgiving was on Thursday and I wanted to go to my family's party.

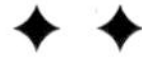

Yes, I was out of my mind, or so my friends and family told me. I had set our family's moving day up for November 22. Had chemotherapy taken place at the three week mark, I would have been moving one day after the infusion. I had caught a lucky break with the doctor agreeing to move me back to four weeks.

Now, make no mistake, I felt decent two weeks out of the month, but I was nowhere near pre-cancer Kim in stamina and ability. I had always used a moving company in my dozen or so moves over the years, but you still have to direct and unpack. The semi pulled down our street at 10 am, and six young men got out. I had a few hundred boxes and eight rooms of furniture plus the garage that had to go. The guys worked fast, but it was a cold and damp November morning and as the hours progressed my strength began to fade. By the time we got to the new house, I was sitting in a chair in the garage trying to direct the guys. Furniture was being set down incorrectly and boxes, even though I had clearly labeled them, were being stacked anywhere there was room.

Having moved numerous times, I had learned label all four sides and top of the box with the room it goes in, with a big black magic marker. Contents were for me to read so it made no difference if they could see it. It started to rain steadily and hard and the guys were just piling; I knew they were making a mess of my house, and I didn't need this aggravation.

I started telling them as they went past me:

"Take that to the basement," or

"Put that in the living room."

Instead they started stacking upstairs boxes in the dining room. The room was wall-to-wall floor-to-ceiling boxes. I walked through the other rooms; they had broken three pieces of my office furniture and loaded up a closet which was supposed to remain at the old house. Obviously, even though I had thought I felt well enough, I wasn't. I had never had these kinds of issues with a moving company, and I had chosen to use one of the largest companies in the country, paying extra, so I wouldn't have problems. However, the Kim I thought I was and the Kim that I actual was became very apparent on that day.

In my head, on the two weeks I wasn't physically getting sick, I knew I wasn't completely myself, but I hadn't realized how bad I had actually become. The weakness in my legs and the fact that multiple trips up and down any staircase in any one day wasn't possible anymore. Plus the standing, I had been standing for about three hours in the early morning, and I was exhausted from it. My mental capacities and my ability to remember things were at an all-time low, and I was too weak to lift anything of substance.

I had physically let myself be taken over by the chemotherapy and done nothing to keep up my stamina or strength. The move was a major eye opener when it came to working out and my condition. I was watching my own father get sicker every month on chemotherapy and I knew he was doing nothing to further his health in the way of diet or exercise. Because I was younger and in better shape physically when I started this processes, I didn't see that I was doing the exact same thing to myself.

I knew something had to change, and it needed to change quickly. The move and all the work that needed to be done was my starting point. I knew that I had done much by packing the house on my own in the past two months. But I had gone slowly, I rested all the time. In the past, I have packed my house in less than a week. As moving day came to a close, Chris and I sat on the couch and visited with our friends Alison and Rich. I felt exhausted and wanted to sleep, but I pushed. I needed my mind to work and keep working instead of letting it shut down like I had been doing for months. I held my own in a conversation with the two of them, and thankfully, they wanted to hang out for a while. I could see Chris getting tired out of the corner of my eye, but I kept myself sharp and sitting upright. The next day, I set the alarm and got up as Chris got ready for work. I drove the Little One to school and started unpacking. I kept up a steady pace until it was time to get Hunter from school. I got up on Thanksgiving and unpacked until I had to head out to see both families for the holiday. Over the holiday weekend, with Chris's help, I decorated the tree and the rest of the house for Christmas. I pushed myself as hard as I could, and on Monday, I showed up for chemotherapy bright and early, knowing that my home was unpacked and I had started the path to physically starting to move my body again, to push myself everyday instead of sitting on the couch.

I felt better about myself in general than I had in months. I was having an 'up' week and I thought once again I had the power and determination to beat this and get myself into yet another remission.

"Gosh, I wish there was something good I could say about chemotherapy. But I hate every minute of it."

- Tom R.
2 year chemotherapy patient

CHAPTER THIRTY-ONE
WHAT'S A NEUTROPHIL?

I showed up at the hospital the following Monday with my youngest sister Jennifer and The Other. During my first go-round in 2010, Chris's mom had taken me to my first three chemo treatments. The last three I was accompanied by my sister Michaelene, then my girlfriend Danielle and, for my final treatment, Chris. I was going on treatment number five for this round, and for the first four, Chris's mom had taken me. It was time to let her rest which meant getting other people to drive me and then sit there all day. Danielle was the obvious choice. She had volunteered to do it and knew what to expect having gone through it all with her son. However, we were getting close to the holidays, and she was a wife, mother, and worked full-time. I wanted to save that resource for after the first of the year. In addition to those caretakers, there was a whole network of people in my case, friends and family who helped me, physically, financially and emotionally. I was very lucky in that respect; most people have only one or two people. I had several stepping up.

Selecting someone to help you through cancer, (or what the industry that cancer has become calls 'a caretaker') is a little bit of luck, a lot of love, and some patience and common sense.

I watched and listened when it came to my caretakers. My sister Michaelene said it best right after my surgery and the start of my chemotherapy. She arrived at our home with homemade apple dumplings, a gallon of fruit punch, and a large cola slushy.

"I don't know what to do… so I did what I know how to do… bake you your favorite apple dumplings, bring you Hawaiian Punch, 'cause I know it's a favorite from childhood, and here's a cola slushy."

It was what I needed at the moment. Someone who made it about what I needed or liked not about the hardship it presented on them. Michaelene hadn't made homemade apple dumplings for years. I knew why—because they were a pain in the ass to make! Yet she did it because she knew I loved them! I didn't have to ask; she took it upon herself. Her regular weekly supermarket shopping didn't include the kid's drinks aisle, because she had no kids, and yet she wheeled her cart down the aisle and picked up the largest container she could find of the fruit punch. There was no convenience store that sold slushies on the way to our house, my brother-in-law drove out of his way to find one around my house and bring it to me. That's how they both rolled. I never heard a word about it either. By a word I mean throwing it in my face to hurt me or the ones I loved. I started to get that kind of response from other people as I got farther into my treatment

"Hey, I helped you do this. How come you can't…"

From people I couldn't believe would do such a thing. I started to see patterns forming with individuals; my cancer became their burden to complain to people about and hold over my head when they didn't get what they wanted or felt un-included.

This became a sore spot with me. I thought I was selecting my caregivers carefully. People I felt I could be open and honest with on all accounts. I never wanted my closest confidants to know my bathroom routines; however, it became necessary as time went on.

The cancer you are dealt is for you alone to cope with. It is all you can do to keep from worrying on a daily basis about everyone and everything. What you don't need to do is worry about a caretaker and what their reaction is going to be to your every move. Make no mistake, the job of a caretaker is no picnic; they get to cart your ass around everywhere and wait. They have to sit with you during your most down and destructive moments trying to keep you uplifted and focused. Some people have the best intentions but in the end are not equipped to handle all the emotions required for your benefit. Others are capable of helping but only in small doses or in very specific ways. For as much as you have on your mind, it is important to keep all these people straight and what their capabilities are, and don't be afraid to push back. After overhearing someone talk to Chris in a very derogatory way when he didn't do what they wanted, I was furious and done with that person. I learned something very important from a friendship lost that day—my health and my emotional well-being are more important to me than any one person.

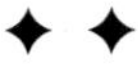

I checked in that November morning late with my number one caretaker Chris. My sister Jennifer also wanted to be there. She had brought along a digital video recorder. She followed me through all the steps and while I was waiting for the meds to be sent from the pharmacy, she and I walked around the facility. She saw how many people were waiting for treatment. That morning was like so many others; the waiting room was overflowing and people were sitting in the hallways adjacent to the waiting room. Wheelchairs lined the wall and caregivers paced around without a place to sit except the floor. We settled for a seat in the library, and Jennifer started reading some of the material that was available. I pointed out the discrepancies in money division. The two new clinics on the other side of the library gleamed compared to the older lab and infusion center. As we looked out of the library windows, we noticed that the breast cancer clinic looked like an entrance to a hotel and nobody was sitting on the floor. We were at about the seventy-five minute mark when I decided we should walk back toward the lab. The light-up beeper they give you still hadn't gone off, and I was getting impatient. The waiting room had only gotten worse. We lucked out and farther down the hall were three open chairs. We sat down to wait when the senior couple next to me started a conversation.

Turns out they were driving in over a hundred miles to come to this cancer hospital. He was eight years into colon cancer and had never been off chemo. They thought by coming here he might get a newer or better treatment than the small center he had been going to in the southern part of the state. They did try newer things, only to put him back on what he had been receiving originally, that treatment kept the cancer cells from spreading and made him less sick than the new treatments. I took the chance and asked about his side-effects.

"Oh they are rough for sure."

I looked at the elderly gentleman's wife. Knowing that these people were more than a full generation older than me, he might not be so forthcoming and blunt, but I needed to try.

"How rough?" I asked her.

"I'm not really sure," she paused and grabbed his hand. *"He makes me stay at my sister's for four days a month. You know, during the worst of it, I guess."*

I looked at the gentleman and nodded in a knowing way, *"That bad?"*

"I had dysentery when serving in the army, I would gladly take that every day for the rest of my life over chemo side-effects."

"I feel your pain! Why do you make your wife leave? I make that one help me." I said glancing back at Chris.

"Oh, she has enough to do and worry about. The way I figure it, I can still get around and clean up after myself so it gives her a little break and I try to sleep as much as I can. We've been married for over fifty years, and I feel like she doesn't need to see THAT.*"*

She interjected, *"Oh yeah, he cleans up."* She winked at me. *"It does scare me from time to time. Once, I actually thought he had died. The bathroom and every surface was covered in… well, you know…"* She looked down, her cheeks turning a light shade of pink.

Our conversation was interrupted by the nurse who put the IV into my port walking up to us. She looked directly at me.

"If you see me again, it's not good. Come on back with me." She turned to walk back to the lab.

I got up from my chair, raised an eyebrow to Chris, and followed the nurse back into the infusion center. She stopped walking at the nurse's station that was at the back of the infusion center.

"I've already called the doctor. We are moving your chemo back one week because your baby neutrophils are too low."

"What's a neutrophil?"

"It's the small white blood cells that form to make your larger white cells." She handed me a piece of paper with all my numbers on it. I noticed the white neutrophils number was circled and there was an 'L' next to the number.

"So much for the Kale," I said.

"Kale?" the nurse asked.

"Yeah, when they said my white count was low and I had to come back for the Neulasta shot I researched food that naturally builds white counts. Kale came up as the biggy."

I had, in my ultimate wisdom, tried to start eating better by upping my vegetable intake. When I learned how incredibly good kale was for you, I added two cups a day to my diet. I put it in everything and made salads of it. I cooked it, baked it, and ate it fresh. However, with this news, I wasn't sure if this process did any good or not. Every book on cancer I had read touted the ways of vegetables and being a vegetarian. I had done just that over the last month. Only my counts were lower than they had ever been.

"Well, it can't hurt; can you imagine your counts without the shot and vegetables? You'd be way lower." The nurse pointed to a chart with the normal range and then to my number. I was a tenth of a point under. *"We will have you wait a week and come back, then we'll draw blood and hopefully that will work, and you will only be a week late on your treatment."*

"And if it doesn't go up?"

"Then, we wait another week," she said flatly. *"But hopefully that doesn't happen."* She started to address a woman sitting in front of a computer at the nurse's station but dressed in street clothes.

"We need to set up Kim for a week from today for infusion."

"What about my other appointments that are already scheduled? Moving this back, messes them up," I interjected.

The woman at the counter said, *"I can fix all of those and print you a new calendar."*

The nurse stood there and talked about the kale and other vegetables to eat while the woman adjusted all my appointments. Once I was handed a calendar, she sat me in the nearest open chair and removed the IV.

"You are all set. We'll see you next week!" She said to me.

I exited the infusion center and returned to where Jennifer and Chris were waiting. I was disappointed in myself for not eating healthy enough to keep my counts in the normal range. I was also bummed because Jennifer had taken time away from work to come out here, and they were sending me home.

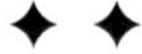

I went home and started researching foods to help build my white counts. I also started to reread the chapters in all the cancer books that had been given to me about diet. I had read all of them, but because I was looking for other information at the time, I mostly discounted what they had to say.

The books were all very similar in their message: 'diet and exercise' will help. It was only the severity at which they thought people should change their lifestyles that they differed. The other problem with the books was that they all addressed different cancers than mine. But, I re-read each of them anyway, concentrating this time on the diet end of the conversations. I also starting tapping into my friends who were vegetarians and vegans, not so much as to what they ate but what they knew about nutrition content in fruits and vegetables as well as whole grains.

I found many people to be vegetarians on principle because they were against the treatment that animals received in the processing role of food production. Not really what I was looking for. Their diets were high in processed foods without meats, white flour products like pasta and especially cheese, none of which were of any benefit to me. Vegans were so severe in there concepts that it left out other things I would need–like bigger quantities of proteins. Frankly, I felt there was room in my life for a little bit of eggs and dairy.

I had upped my water intake since the stent surgery. That surgery required at least two quarts of water a day. I had started out good on fresh-brewed green tea with a whole fresh lemon juiced into a pitcher. But I had gotten lazy about keeping up with the process; I was not getting my thirty-two ounces a day, opting most times for the easier soda-pop.

My vegetable intake was good but not great. I managed at dinner to get a salad in along with a few serving of vegetables, but my remission consumption of a full eight-to-ten servings a day was long gone. Fruit was limited to the occasional orange or apple. I had only just added kale for the white counts, but I was sure without the other vegetables, I wasn't making much progress.

I really didn't want to be that person. I had no desire to eat nothing but vegetables, fruit and whole grains. In fact, I wasn't a big fan of whole grain. I would opt for white bread or pasta any day over a whole grain.

I knew my life depended on at least a bit of an effort on my part. So, I reluctantly headed off to the store to stock up on not just fruits and vegetables but fish. I had read that fish might help with zinc which in turn could raise the white counts especially the neutrophils. Of course, me being, me that meant the only real fish I liked was albacore tuna fish. I ate it every day for lunch and a kale salad for dinner. I dug out the only oatmeal I would eat, an old favorite from when I was a kid, and added an apple with it for breakfast. I tried to cook every day for dinner instead of using the prepackaged things that were sitting in the freezer, which I had turned to after years of never eating if only for their convenience while I was sick.

I made some other changes regarding chemicals also. I had read way back when all this started in one of the books about a woman who after contracting cancer eliminated all chemicals from her life. She started by one day listing all the chemicals in everything she used or ate. At the end of the day, she had over three thousand items. She looked each one up and anything that wasn't natural or organic, she stopped using or eating. I tried that one morning, and the list was so long after getting ready to go to work that I stopped, but it made me think twice about certain things. I stopped using nail polish and nail polish remover because of the chemicals. I looked twice at the cleaners I used around the house and found some of the best things were the basics like name brand window cleaner and a baking soda based bathroom cleaner. I got rid of all the other products. I thought about all the things that I had done in my life not thinking twice about where I would be taking in chemicals, either by breathing them, placing them on my body or eating them. Should I have been more careful? I couldn't fix the past, but I could watch what I did in the future. My biggest opponent? Me! That's correct; I had no one opposing me except me. Although I knew what was probably best for my health, and to treat my cancer was to change many things about my lifestyle such as the products I used and the way I ate. I actually liked all the conveniences that were at my disposal. I used them daily, always had, and I had never really bought into the assumption that all these things caused cancer. I felt everything I had done was in moderation, with the exception of my enormous consumption of caffeine-based products for the two years preceding my diagnosis. Therefore, convincing me I had to change everything about who I was, was unfortunately, going to be a battle with myself.

"You learn really fast those who truly love you and genuinely want to help, and those who do it for the attention and to hold the fact that they help over your head."

\- Kim Henderly

CHAPTER THIRTY-TWO

IT WILL BE A MIRACLE IF HE GETS THROUGH THIS

As the next round of treatment approached, I was at my wit's end and on the cusp of another remission, and I started to feel the emotional toll it was taking on me now. I didn't enter the treatment in an upbeat state of mind but a more negative one. I didn't want to deal with the extra side-effects the Neulasta I assumed had caused, and I was sick of the twelve-day constipation battle.

The thought in this round was to get me off the Nuelasta. So, that meant getting up the white counts with food. I did my due diligence filling up on dark kale, dark green veggies, garlic, and black pepper. I used a soup base that a friend had provided to help with constipation during the treatments and made many of my meals of this vegetarian soup with the added vegetables and spices.

Then, for the second time since I was diagnosed with cancer, my brand new stove broke.

So much for cooking down all these veggies!

What was going on with me? I couldn't believe my luck. You start to think that your number is up even though you don't want it to be but the signs are everywhere. The stuff that used to fall into place no longer does; things go wrong more often. I found myself more on the couch and less on my feet. I was floundering in my own world with no sense of what I was supposed to do.

Worried daily that my bowels would perforate from not being able to go for a week at a time.

Worried that nobody would be here when something went terribly wrong.

Worried that I would lie in a bed in this new home that didn't feel like mine as a parade of people came to say goodbye as I lay dying.

I worried about who would take care of My Other. I wanted to go on loving him, protecting him from the idiots out there that wanted to cause him emotional harm, taking care of him. Yet, I knew I had to relinquish all that. It was weighing on my psyche.

That round of infusion came following the Thanksgiving break. Too many sick people were jammed into a room–waiting for the people to get to work following a holiday off. As a man in his mid-twenties was wheeled up next to where I was sitting and began to vomit into a waste basket, I knew I was in for a long ride. I got up and moved to the outer waiting room, looking closely at the faces of the men and women who graced every spare seat, not only in the waiting room, but the hallway. There wasn't an open chair or wall-space to lean against. Frustration bled into the air.

There were no Lance Armstrongs, no Farrah Faucetts; the chick from E news who couldn't have a baby and was diagnosed with early stages of breast cancer didn't come here. I was sitting in one of the supposed "top cancer centers in the country" and looking around at the slow death that was prevailing everywhere. People, un-showered and in dirty clothes, coughed uncontrollably, spreading things like the common cold which could kill the person harboring cancer. There were no TV's here, no bright peppy people, just a lot of sad workers back too soon from their well-deserved holiday breaks, who were trained to say "hi" or "good morning" politely to everyone they came in contact with. It was a disgusting display of our American Healthcare System. Not because it was underfunded but because I watched the heavily-funded breast clinic people and the men going into the clinic funded by a local baseball hero being treated so much better. beautiful new facilities with plenty of room for all the patients to sit, you never saw a breast cancer patient or their caregiver sitting on the floor in the hall vomiting into a garbage can. As the rest of us with the terminal cancers were left to fend for themselves in one small, old waiting room, waiting for hours for the pharmacist to show up and send up the meds.

That day I arrived at 8:05 for an 8:15 chemo infusion. I got to my bed for the infusion at 10:20 and still sat there for another twenty minutes. It was ridiculous! On top of all that, the fire marshal and the health department were making their appointed rounds. I felt bad for the nurses. Overworked and now being told to shut doors and move things out of the way. Instead of answering the alarms on the IVs, they were bothering the few volunteers that they do have about how their lunch carts were set up. Having worked hospitality for twenty-three years, there was nothing wrong with the carts, other than it wasn't the way that particular health inspector wanted it on that particular day. They slowed down the process and upset the volunteers. The volunteers needed by the sick people.

Many of the people that come to these centers don't have help. They call for rides or get dropped off alone. The friendly words of the volunteers are all they have. Like I said, these aren't the rich and famous; these are the ordinary lower and middle-class people. Sure, you'd like to take your mom, or your sister, or grandmother or friend for treatment, but it's a several hour process on a monthly basis or perhaps even weekly or daily basis. It sucks. People have their own families to take care of, they have jobs, lives. It's hard to get someone to sit for seven to nine hours every three or four weeks (or once a week in some cases).

No... Farrah and her girlfriend don't come here. Just the people that Medicaid and Medicare have deemed worthy enough for treatment or those lucky enough to have a spouse still employed with insurance. I dread the day that my insurance would end. It always does–there is always a reason when this much money is being spent. Then, at that point, I know that death won't be but months behind me.

We all fight so hard for this small part of existence. Wanting to stay here with the ones we love so dearly. Worried for their future, jealous of what will happen without our presence. It's a never-ending cycle this thing we call cancer. The worry, the fear, the unknown, the constant thought that what you deemed was controllable is actually spiraling into the unknown. No one can feel like you. No one can understand.

As I got sicker, I felt that people needed to come around more. It's like driving by a traffic accident.

Personally, I always made it a point not to look. It seemed so invasive, so rude. Yet, car after car would slow down and get a good look at the tragedy that was unfolding.

It felt that way with my illness. People volunteered to 'assist' me yet only on the days that I was vomiting uncontrollably or couldn't move because of the pain like they wanted to wear my pain as a badge of honor on 'how they were helping me.'

It was disgusting, and yet when I physically needed some help I got a lot of–

"Well, I can be there in a few hours..."

" I have to stop here and go pick up some things..." and

"I haven't had my coffee yet."

I was at my wits' end, and nobody seemed to comprehend any of this. I was at a loss of how to get my point across.

The insurance company had approved the Avastin. I was relieved and scared about what side-effects were going to be thrown at me next. I asked for the sheet listing side-effects. As soon as I read the sheet, I knew I was in for trouble.

"In about 30% of the people," glared back from the top of the page.

Yeah, that was way too high a number for it not to affect me, and as the days went on following the infusion, they crept in one at a time. First, it was a little itchy nose that turned into blowing my nose and having snot come out, to blowing my nose and having blood. I was worried. I could handle that, but I didn't want to end up with an all-out nosebleed at work, in a store, or at a friend's house. People would totally freak! ARGH! I hated when I over thought things!

After the itchy nose, came the headache. A spot on the very top of my head on the left side a little towards the back would throb randomly. If I pressed on it for a minute, it seemed to subside for that moment. It came and went, and I thought 'well if that's it, I can handle it.' Then came Monday morning, eight days after receiving the drug, I woke to a familiar feeling. My chest had some pressure and felt cold. It wasn't painful to breathe in. It just wasn't normal.

Upper respiratory infection.

It was one of the listed side-effects. When I saw it, I thought 'oh great another pill to take.' I'm not opposed to antibiotics. I wanted every white blood cell I had fighting this cancer, not some other stupid infection, an infection by the way that I had no reason to have. I hadn't been anywhere public (other than the cancer center, and I wore a mask and gloves). The Other and I had holed up in the living room for the past week. He was a nut at work disinfecting everything and hand-washing, then changing his clothes when he came home and showering. No, this infection was low-grade and there simply because of the Avastin.

I was in a quandary now. It was Monday, and I knew that the cancer center would have them stacked to the ceiling. I wasn't feeling up to driving myself downtown anyways. Should I wait this out, or should I ask for an antibiotic? Would they insist on seeing me? Would they tell me to go to urgent care, or worse yet *my primary care physician*, which I didn't have. I sat there on that Monday feeling the respiratory infection take hold.

I thought when that infection came I was through the side-effects but like clockwork on Monday afternoon the chills started like last month. A few hours later I was vomiting uncontrollably again. This time, I was positive it was the shot to build the white blood cells.

I had been trying to force myself to do things around the house but found myself in bed more and more. I didn't have the mental mindset going into this round to hold myself up high and the side-effects were winning. I stopped following the diet with more vegetables and drinking green tea. I ate and drank what made me happy: junk food and pop. I had no desire to help myself. I wanted this all to be over and be in another remission. Last go-round I would have been looking at one more round but not this time. I knew my number was still too high.

I was sick of being sick all the time. Winter had set in again and the only thing that ever made me feel better was the two days I went into work and the weekends when Chris was with me all the time. I knew I was close to an emotional break of some type and I wanted to stop it but didn't know how. I took to the couch on most days, not moving around much. I had tried even doing some painting but when that second round of effects hit I was depressed over it. Two full weeks of being sick was not cutting it for me and there was no end in sight.

My side-effect list was also increasing by the day. I had added the receding gums, as well as the nosebleed and headaches, and add to it the extra day of chills and vomiting. You would think that's where it would stop, but no.... the numbness in my hands and feet had spread. Instead of the small circle on my foot and the tips of the index finger and thumb, it had taken over all my toes and both my thumbs as well as the first two fingers on both hands including the palms and soles of my feet. Of course, not knowing any better at the time, I went outside in the cold without my hands and feet well protected. It caused an uncontrollable itching in the parts that were numb. I was ready to scratch my skin right off! I found another thread on-line of people talking about the itching and determined it to be another side-effect.

The list of what I was suffering through was growing ever longer, and I was upset, angry and drained. I wanted so much to fight on, but I was losing my will to fight quickly. I started qualifying my own death in my head yet I kept coming back to the same things:

Chris and Hunter. If it wasn't for the two of them, I would have let go at that point. I had been through enough. I was tired and felt defeated by the system of healthcare and its treatment of cancer patients. I felt like I kept screaming about it and, at this point, people were sick of hearing me complain.

On top of feeling sorry for myself, the week before Christmas sent my father into the hospital. He had been on chemotherapy for over three years now, fighting the Multiple Myeloma within him, and he was fighting pneumonia on top of it.

It was this past Easter when my dad's health issues had multiplied. A bout with pneumonia and issues with breathing had sent him to the hospital. After the doctors in the ER had admitted him, it had been discovered that he was in congestive heart failure. I had been furious with his not one, but two, cardiologists that he had been seeing. How the hell did they miss that?! The weeklong stay in the hospital had gotten him back on his feet but never quite the same. It was an issue for him to walk, to drive. I didn't know what was getting the better of him the cancer, its treatment, or now this heart issue. The admittance in the third week of December was scary.

The nimrod doctor said to my mom right after he was admitted, *"It will be a miracle if he makes it though this."*

I didn't like my dad's cancer center; it was part of the original network that had sent me packing to find 'a general surgeon' after finding 'the mass.' I wasn't impressed with the heart doctors or the oncologist. They were like the hospital I had left, always following protocol and not treating the patient for who they are.

The texts and phone calls were coming in from my sisters. Luckily, I was almost done with side-effects and thought I could make the drive out to see him the next morning.

I was worried about my feet, the numbness, and being able to make the hour plus drive with two major expressway changes.

The numbness was an odd feeling, not quite like pins and needles or your foot falling asleep. You could feel your foot but from the inside not the outside. When you took a step, it felt like your foot was hitting two inches above the ground. Strap on to your foot something light-weight but sturdy, like a piece of Styrofoam packing that's about 3-4 inches thick, and then try to walk around the living room. At first, it will feel weird and then the tripping and sticking will start as you get used to it. Yet, remember you adapt but your footing doesn't change. So, there is a definite issue with driving, such as—are you pressing on the accelerator too much or too little?

I decided to take the longer route which would keep me out of heavy traffic and expressway interchanges. I would take my time and people could go around me if they didn't like it.

My dad didn't look like he was at Death's door. He was dozing when I came in with my sister. He got up a bit after that and ate. I was pleased that he was feeling a bit better but I was not pleased at the hospital surroundings. My dad told me the lady in the next room had been up all night screaming for help and his IV alarm was going off every fifteen minutes. I knew how to reset the IV from my own experiences and my sister kept hitting reset to shut off the alarm. I asked the nurse why it was going off, and she said he needed to keep his arm straight. They had placed the IV in the fold of his arm. I called the person who did that an idiot and asked for it to be changed. She assured me there was only a half hour left on the antibiotic and then he would be done. I only stayed for a short time as my mom showed up, and my dad wanted her around—not all of us girls who had shown up to see him because of the doctor's words to my mom.

A couple of days later, it was Christmas Eve and I made my way back to the hospital. This time Chris drove me. We got there, and my sister Michaelene and her husband Ken were already visiting. The alarm was going off, and the lady in the next room was still yelling. I asked my dad who now looked like he hadn't slept in days if these things had been constant. He said yes someone or the alarm was waking him up all night long. I lost it. All the things I had wanted to yell about in the problems with my own care got manifested at the nurses and aides sitting at the nurse's station.

"WHAT THE HELL IS GOING ON HERE? I was here two days ago and my dad's IV alarm was going off and the lady in the next room was screaming for help. He is supposed to be resting! Now fix the IV, and either help the lady, move the lady, or move my dad!"

The four of them looked at each other stunned. One said his room number to the other.

"Oh right, well he has to keep his arm straight."

"BULLSHIT!!" I screamed as I lifted the sleeve on my shirt. On my previous chemo treatment, I had the girl draw blood from my arm, not my port, and the bruise was still there.

"They poke me all the time and I can move and waive my arms around…" I was flailing both arms in the air like a mad woman *"…and the alarm never goes off! FIX IT NOW!!"*

It was obvious I was a cancer patient. Bald head, no eyebrows or eyelashes. I hadn't said chemo, but they knew what I was talking about. They called for my dad's nurse who immediately said,

"He'll have to wait. I'm busy."

I looked over at the board. Because of the holiday, this nurse had way too many patients and so did the one aide that I saw running around. I felt my blood pressure rising and I knew being this upset wasn't good for me, but I sure in the hell wasn't going to let this go. I had enough to deal with, and I wasn't ready to deal with my dad's death because the hospital decided he was too sick to care about.

"If she is too busy," I said with all the sarcasm I could manage. *"Then find the dipshit nurse supervisor who didn't schedule enough people. Tell her to push her fat ass away from her family's dinner table and get in here and help my dad because this will be a very uncomfortable night for everyone*

working unless this is fixed NOW!"

While I was ranting, they had paged someone else. A new nurse came scurrying down the hall. The girls behind the desk told her the problem. She said she would take care of it herself and we walked back to my dad's room. She started a new IV farther up his arm and while doing that asked him why he was so bruised up.

My dad said sarcastically, *"Ask the people who work here and take my blood every five minutes."*

I knew it was an exaggeration, but he was right. Both arms were bruised from the wrist to the elbow. It was unnecessary and laziness on the phlebotomist's part.

This new nurse not only fixed the IV but got my dad into a new room away from the screaming woman. I thanked her and explained that I hated to be so mean, but I was here two days ago and the same things were going on and that he couldn't get better if he couldn't rest.

My dad got the rest and antibiotics he needed, and came out of it. If you believed the original ER doctor's coincidental and prophetic pronouncement: 'a miracle.' I think it was common sense and medicine. When I visited him again after Christmas, my mom told me he needed a shower and hadn't had one since he had checked in five days ago. Oh man, time to bring 'Mean Kim' out again. My mom needed a break and I told her I would sit with my dad and see that a shower was ordered. It was my good fortune that a social worker stopped by to check on my dad while I was sitting there. She wanted to wake him up to ask him questions; I had already sent away three people trying to get into his room to 'check on him.' I let her in and she woke my dad. He answered all her stupid questions and asked if he needed anything.

He said no, and I spoke up,*"he needs help taking a shower."*

The social worker glanced down at the papers in her lap and said, *"Oh, he's hooked to oxygen so they can't give him a shower. He will pass out from lack of oxygen."*

I wanted to laugh out loud at the stupidity of that statement. I withheld my laughter and resorted to my usual sarcasm, looked her right in the eye, and said:

"Let me get this straight. Because he will be on oxygen now for the rest

of his life, he can never shower? Is that what you are telling me?"

I made the statement loud and strong. In effect telling her, you're an idiot and don't feed me a line of shit she responded with:

"No, but the oxygen is attached to the wall.."

Again, an irritating statement to make and I countered:

"So you mean to tell me, in this entire healthcare system, one of the biggest in the state, you don't have a portable oxygen tank you can hook him up to and assist with a shower?"

"Umm… oh yes, we could do that. I will have to ask the doctor, of course."

"Make sure you TELL the doctor his family is insisting on a shower by day's end."

"I will do that right now," and with that she got up and hurried out of the room.

My dad laughed.

"You are so mean! They don't want me to have a shower 'cause people slip and sue the hospital."

"Are you gonna sue the hospital Dad?"

"No."

"Then they need to help you take a shower."

I ordered lunch for my dad, and he took a nap until my mom returned and a friend stopped by to visit.

Why bring up all this? For two reasons:

The first is the friend that stopped in while having a casual conversation with him and my mom as my dad ate his lunch he said, *"When I was in the hospital, I wondered why people came to visit and talked to each other and not to me."*

Before he made the statement, I thought to myself, does my dad really want this guy here? He is half-dressed, not feeling well, and this is a neighbor sauntering in here not immediate family. I took offence to what he said. I was talking to keep the conversation going and keep this guy entertained while my dad ate, and he was letting me know that he came to talk to my dad. I thought about my own stay in the hospital. I had talked to most of my visitors. However, when Alison had come to see me, I was in the middle of some of the worst of it, and I had been tired. I was so grateful that my parents were also visiting, and she and my dad had sat and talked while I dozed on and off. I had tried staying awake to talk but couldn't. I know it made Alison more comfortable to have someone to talk to.

I think if it is your intention to go to the hospital and have a meaningful conversation with someone, you can't be upset if they are not on your timeframe for conversation. If you are prepared to see someone in a state of undress and illness and you know for a fact that the person is ok with you seeing them like that, then, it is ok to visit.

I never went to see Andrea or Karen in the hospital because I knew what our relationship was, and I was comfortable with that. Everyone has to make their own choice, but you must consider the person you are seeing. Remember you are going there for them, not to appease yourself in some way.

The second and very important reason I bring up this incident is what it did for me and what it made me understand.

Going into all of this, I was down. Thinking of someone else besides myself gave me the kick I needed to rebound out of what could have turned into full blow depression. I also found my voice again and used it to speak up for my dad. Although I had tried several times to speak up for myself, I didn't seem to be as effective at getting what I needed for me.

My dad is a smart man and working for the medical examiner's office for all those years gave him medical knowledge that most don't possess. I found myself doing what he did in my own care. Not questioning the medical staff enough, not being loud enough, and not speaking up for myself. When I did, I had been met with resistance at the last hospital. I knew I needed to keep this in the back of my mind at all times so that my care would be top-of-the-line and in my best interest no matter what.

CHAPTER THIRTY-THREE
THE SHEATH

I made it through the rest of the holidays, celebrating with my sisters and brother-in-laws. The holidays falling on weekends helped. Chris was around a lot more. He was not working because of the holiday when chemo number six rolled around on the New Year's weekend.

I usually was scheduled to see the doctor the day of chemo. This appointment was made without the doctor's visit. There were very few people even in the hospital and some areas were closed off. Labs were at 7:30, and by 8:30 I was back in my room hooked up to the IV. Jennifer came again with the video camera and asked questions about the facility and what was being administered to me. My alarm only went off when the IV was done and the nurse showed up within seconds. She then understood why I was so annoyed with our dad's alarm.

Nobody mentioned the Neulasta shot, and I didn't ask. I looked at my numbers and they were the same number as before when they told me I had to have the shot. I kept my mouth shut.

I went through the same horrible side-effects as usual only I felt like they were getting worse and taking longer.

Chris told me everything was happening in the same order, for the same length of time, and what seemed like the same intensity. I, on the other hand, felt like they were getting away from me. I couldn't get out of bed for eight days. I barely ate, and what I did eat was junk food. Drinking water made me vomit, so I only drank pop. And, in an effort to try and combat the ever worsening constipation, I had started on the recommended over-the-counter laxative mixed with apple cider two days before chemo. I had pooped a small amount on December 31st in the morning and chemo was on January 2nd. Until I started vomiting on Sunday night January 8th, I hadn't taken a shit. Nine days. It was the longest I had gone, without even a little hard stool that I had to pull out myself. Nothing. I had taken the OTC laxative faithfully every morning hoping that it would help. I was petrified. I felt like my bowels were shutting down.

After vomiting uncontrollably for more than fifteen minutes, I felt my stomach starting to turn and I knew what was coming. I sat down on the toilet and grabbed the bucket. Shit poured out of me in huge clumps. Our toilet from the 1960's couldn't keep up and refill fast enough. I had to figure out how to change, to shit in the bucket and puke in the toilet. I knew my stomach contents were almost out. I stood up to make the move. Nope that wasn't gonna work. I was scared of the toilet overflowing. I flushed as often as it would allow me. I caught a break about fifteen minutes later. I needed a shower but had no energy to stand in the shower. I had Chris put towels on the bed. I went to lie down and cry.

"This is worse than ever before."

He tried to assure me that it wasn't. Yet, I could feel it. My body wasn't recovering as well as it needed to, and it was getting harder to take the punishment of the barrage of side-effects I was being hit with. My nose was now in even worse shape. Every time I would blow it, there was more and more blood. Both my husband and Charlotte had had to have their noses cauterized from nosebleeds, and I knew I didn't want to have that done. I stopped blowing it and instead used a cotton-tipped swab to carefully extract what was loose. I wanted to try and see if my nose would scab over on its own.

My stomach started to churn and then severe gas pains struck. I went into the bathroom for another round of Kim vs. the toilet and bucket. When I stood up and looked into the toilet there was blood. Lots of it. Bright red. I kept thinking: don't panic; don't panic. My ass was on fire. I reached under the cabinet for the baby salve and used it. It burned more. I was hoping the burning meant I broke a hemorrhoid and nothing more.

I lay down again. The processes went on throughout the night until there was nothing left in me. The blood slowed down too. The next day, I googled bright-red blood while having a bowel movement.

It posted as one of two things, a hemorrhoid or an anal fissure. I crossed my fingers and hoped for the 'roid.

This was going to be a hard call to the doctor, and had I not been through enough embarrassing things, but now someone was going to have to check my asshole. I couldn't bring myself to make the call. I crawled under the covers and went to sleep instead. The week went on and every day I felt a little better. Without the shot, I didn't have the round of chills or a second vomiting incident. Now, I was sure that the white booster shot is what caused that second round of vomiting.

What most people don't know or don't realize is that life still goes on, and the body deteriorates at a more rapid rate. The aging process is accelerated as the chemotherapy drugs destroy good and bad reproducing cells. You aren't the same person physically after eight treatments compared to the first couple. Therefore, every month, chemo side-effects become more and more magnified.

A major worry on the list of many was the stent placed five months ago, and the date to change it out was fast approaching. Unfortunately, this outpatient procedure, like most, really shouldn't be done if your white counts are low. If I didn't have it changed out, my chances of kidney failure grew. Yet, stopping chemotherapy for about eight weeks could put me on a slippery slope of not being able to control the cancer left to grow for two full months.

Stress was building in me again. I had lost friends to cancer recently. My own father's health was in question. We were just getting by money-wise with me still clinging to my part-time status, and the side-effects seemed to be multiplying and getting worse as I moved forward. I felt the world closing in on me. This doctor didn't think much of the CA125, so I hadn't seen my number in the last few visits. I needed a remission. My body needed a break. I couldn't figure out how my dad had gone through this for three years. I knew by looking at him he was just a part of what he had been physically, from all the treatment.

I was never much for letting things roll off of me; I took everything and everyone to heart. What I had always wanted in my life was a consistent job that I didn't have to worry about getting yelled at every day or losing every time something in the economy went awry and a budget needed to be cut. I didn't want family or friends in turmoil. I wanted everything to be perfect every day, so I could go to sleep happy and content. Of course, I wanted that... but life isn't a 1950's movie with a happy ending now is it?

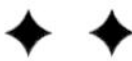

On the last day of January, I headed down to the cancer hospital with my girlfriend Danielle. Again no appointment scheduled with the doctor, but I really didn't feel like I needed to talk to anyone. Chemo amnesia had kicked in, and I had already forgotten the suffering of the last round. Going into round seven, I was in the same place I was with the last hospital. Even though these people listened and tried to help, nobody could really do anything about the side-effects. Every visit to this center, I tried to talk to a different person and ask about their side-effects. I also started asking the women that stopped me in stores to ask about the cancer what they had been through. Everyone had some type of ordeal fairly similar to mine that they never really spoke about .... they just shut everything out of their heads hoping to never have to go through it again. All of them never told a single person how bad it really was.

I was so encouraged by those people who told me they were more than ten years into their survival thanks to the cancer center I was at. It gave me faith that my doctors could get me there also.

My white counts were holding at the same low number as last time, and again, nobody said a word and neither did I. My round of side-effects mirrored the previous month in intensity. I couldn't figure out what to eat or what to do. The blood scared me. The vomiting scared me. I lay in my bed again for eight days too sick to move or do anything else. Barely drinking or eating, I was worried now about the stent. As I came out of it, it was hard to pee, thick and cloudy. I was going a lot more once again. It was like the old days pre-stent when I had to pee six or eight times a night and once an hour during the day. I tried to make up for my lack of water and bad eating on my two good weeks.

The smells that come out of you during side-effects in themselves are enough to make you want to vomit. I pee sometimes and think *'the outhouse in the campgrounds I went to as a kid smelled better than this.'*

✦ ✦

Mid February of 2012, I was sent for another CT scan and five days later a visit with the doctor.

I had been there over ninety minutes between the waiting room and the office; I didn't want to be there but knew I needed to be there. I had to tell the doctor about the Avastin and my nose bleeds. I really wasn't sure if I wanted to continue if there wasn't a reason.

The resident came in first to take notes about what I had to say. I once again complained about the side-effects. When she offered up a suggestion, I laid out the 'been-there-done-that.' I wanted to know the whys and how this was happening. Why all the vomiting with the anti-nausea meds being taken faithfully? She didn't have an answer other than it's the side-effects. I also asked for my CA125.

I felt a bit better after being told the number was down to 82. I qualified it in my head, only a few more treatments and then remission. I couldn't wait to post it on social media again. I felt like I had been posting months of bitching about how hard the side-effects were. I needed to post something positive.

The doctor came in, and I told him I was one Avastin treatment from having my nose cauterized. He immediately said he was taking me off it. That's what I liked about my doctor, no foolin' around. He asked about specific things like the hand and feet numbness. He wasn't happy about that and wanted to take me off the Taxol and put me on Taxotere. I was hesitant. The Taxol was working, and my numbers were way down, but he didn't want the numbness getting worse. In the last round, it had encompassed both my feet completely to the ankle. He said my CT scan looked good and handed me a copy. I didn't have a chance to read the entire thing while he was sitting there, but the thing that caught my eye first was the 4mm nodule was down to 3mm. That hadn't moved since I started chemo, and I thought that the Avastin played a role in its reduction. I wanted to revisit using

Avastin again when I was off chemo to try and get rid of whatever it was.

I listened as the doctor told the nurse what to order for chemo next week. The Carboplatin was still in and they were going to give my twenty-five percent less Taxotere. He looked back at me and said the biggest side-effect with Taxotere is low white counts, and that I was going to have to get the Neulasta shot for sure.

This whole low white count thing was starting to bother me. I had taken the time to look up every word on the sheet they gave me with all my counts. I also lined them up and noticed my counts were at their worst when they had me on a three week spread. I felt like I was rebounding regularly without the shot. To hear that I would have to have it with the Taxotere was not making me a happy camper, but the doctor didn't want me to completely lose feeling in my hands and feet. I wish they were this worried about the fact that I couldn't stop vomiting or my inability to poop during chemo. I was putting my trust in what this guy had to say and his opinions. I had expressed my concerns about changing and he was still fairly certain this was a better move for me.

A week later, I headed down to the cancer center to start the new treatments. My mother-in-law and I had done this so many times we had our routine down. So when I was called to get my IV inserted and blood drawn I really wasn't thinking much about it.

I liked all the nurses in the infusion center. They were happy. I find that when you frequent any place of business often and start to talk to and recognize people they get comfortable and start complaining, especially about work. That didn't happen here. At the other hospital, especially in the lab, the girls were always bickering about who was doing more work, their supervisors, and general working conditions and pay. Since I was there a lot and was a talkative person, this opened the door for them to freely talk in front of me and to me about their status at work and how much they hated it. That type of thing never happened here. The staff was always in a good mood, and I liked that. You know that life doesn't really deal everyone a perfect day. However, this group of people left their crap at the door in order to put a good spin on the patients' crappy day. Even though I liked all the nurses, a couple really stuck out as my favorites, with my original nurse being at the top of the list. That day, I was called by another girl who was at the top of my like list. She reminded me of my friend Megan. Because she not only looked like a curly brunette version of my blonde friend, but she had this little twinkle in her eye that made me think she had the same kind of off-color humor that Megan possessed when she was not working. She always made me laugh when she had to put in my IV or had to administer the white blood cell booster shot. Today was no different.

When she called my name, and I came walking back, she said:

"I saw your name and knew this was going to be easy!" she said to me with a smile.

"Yes, I'm a big no to all questions and let's-move-it-along kinda girl."

"I like that!"

I sat in her chair, and she took my vitals. My blood pressure was a little higher than normal. I answered all the questions with my usual 'No's' and it was on to insert the IV. She couldn't get a blood draw. When I entered the nurses' room a few minutes before, I had noticed a woman in the corner chair, feet in the air and head closest to the floor, with two nurses standing over her; I had never seen that before and had no idea what they were doing to her.

"Come on," the nurse said talking to my IV.

Recently, (to be exact during the past four blood draws) I had listened to the nurses make comments about the blood coming out slow for the draw. They all ended up getting what they needed, but it took a few minutes. This time there was no blood coming out. I was asked to put my hands over my head. That didn't work. Then, I was being inverted like the woman I had just seen. Neither thing worked and it started to make me a little nervous. I didn't want chemo going into a vein. Teri had that done, and she said she used to hide her arms after a while.

My nurse explained everything as she went along.

Ports can form a 'sheath' over them which will prevent the blood flow. She injected some medicine to break it up and ordered another drug from the pharmacy. She told me that sometimes the first medicine will break up the sheath, and I wouldn't need the second medicine. I asked if it was common to have this happen. She told me that it just really depends on the person and their body. Some never have it form. Some have to be injected with these meds all the time; and some might have it happen once and then never again. They waited several minutes and tried again. No luck. So, the second medicine was injected. Then, I had to wait an hour for the medicine to work before they could try again. It was back to the waiting room for the hour wait. I sat down frustrated and opened my computer and googled the lack of blood draw. I found threads of recent conversations almost immediately. I also found out quickly how many bad cancer centers, bad nurses and bad doctors there really were out there. One reminded me of the oncology nurse I had come in contact with at the previous hospital. Telling the woman who started the thread after she questioned the lack of blood draw from the port,

"She didn't know what she was talking about, and that they didn't HAVE to draw blood from her port. Her port was for medicine to go INTO her body, and if she had to get blood drawn from her arm, then too bad for her."

The tone of that thread and the people who posted under it reminded me over and over again how I needed to always speak up for myself. As I came to realize, dozens upon dozens of people were telling this woman, *"If that's what they told you, go with it, and don't worry, they know what they are doing."* When you read something like that, it makes you scared. Here was someone asking for help, and tons of people told her *'accept the circumstances, don't question.'* Each one was incorrect. I was happy when I read farther down the thread because there were a couple who spoke up, explained the 'sheath' and procedurally the same thing I was now going through. I wanted to email the woman and tell her to find a better treatment center, to complain about the nurse and not take any crap, not just blindly accept what they were telling you.

I was starting to understand that there were so many cancer centers out there, and that some were great and some were average. Much of that great or average rating with me truly depended on the knowledge and dedication of the people working within the walls of the center. I also was beginning to understand that absolutely nothing was told to you in advance. If you were lucky enough to be in a great cancer center, then as things came up, you would be privy to information as the staff explained what was going on. If you ended up in one of the cancer centers that were getting by on protocol, you were likely to receive sporadic, sub-standard care and misinformation.

I wanted to email the people in the threads who weren't getting the correct answers for something like a sheath. Especially one gentleman I read a comment from, who every time they couldn't draw blood from his port, they replaced it. He was working on his sixth port in four years' time. I thought that was ludicrous and wanted to email him and ask what kind of insurance he had because it seemed excessive and a simple play to make money off him. This is why they state that everyone is different. It's not necessarily the patient that's different. It's the hospital and their knowledge of what needs to be done. Where was all that protocol in these other cancer centers? Shouldn't a clogged port be treated the same way everywhere? Inject the meds; see if the sheath breaks up, and if it doesn't, then discuss other options. I found myself worrying needlessly for the people who had ports and their centers stopped drawing blood from the port when the blood stopped flowing. What would happen to them? It seemed that something like this fell into that category of problems that could easily be avoided.

This one little incident made me realize how much everyone as a whole really didn't know about cancer. With the number of people contracting it broaching the fifty percent mark very quickly, I thought that needed to change. I also counted my blessings that I was able to slowly figure out that I wasn't in a good treatment center. Now having spent the last several months in a good center, the difference was like night and day.

I was sitting at the end of a row of chairs, and Sue got up to get a cup of coffee. I looked up from my computer and over at the person on the other side of where Sue had been sitting.

"Hi, my name is Kim. Do you mind if I ask what type of cancer you have?"

"Not at all. Cervical. This is number ten in my third go-round."

I knew what she meant. The cancer had returned twice after remissions and this was her tenth chemo infusion in that third round.

"Do you have a port?"

"I do. Best thing ever. My mother had breast cancer and didn't have a port. Of course, that was many years ago, but I remember how tender her arms were."

She went on to tell me her story and her mother's. It was joyous and heartbreaking at the same time, and what started out as me fishing to find out if she ever had a sheath brought me back around to my usual questions about her side-effects. She didn't have as many vomiting issues as me, but she showed me her hands after removing her gloves. Her fingernail beds were becoming loose. It was on my top five gross things I have ever seen. She said she was ok with it after watching her mom get so physically ill she thought that her '*dilemma*' was easier to handle. She asked why I didn't wear a wig and gave me a lecture on how I should keep up my appearances as a woman and not let cancer win. I told her I wasn't letting cancer win by exposing its ugly treatment and side-effects to the world.

"More people need to know what we go through," I said to her.

"People would be getting sick themselves if I told them what I went through," she laughed.

"Maybe they need to?" I responded.

"Oh honey, I have all boys. I would be way too embarrassed to share that with any of them."

There it was again; cover it up, and don't let anyone know what is happening to you because it's embarrassing.

At exactly an hour, another nurse came to get me. As I walked back into the nurse's room, I saw the lady who had been inverted.

"Sorry. It started with me and then I passed it on!" she joked.

I smiled. *"I saw you when I came in and was wondering what they were doing. That's what I get for being nosy!"*

I turned to the nurse and asked, *"Now what if this doesn't work?"*

"Then, we do it again until it does."

"Seriously? Does that happen a lot?"

"A lot? No, but it happens. I've seen people take up to three rounds."

And then my favorite nurse piped in, *"But I have faith, this will work. I thought it would work after the first injection."*

They both smiled as the nurse who was helping me said:

"Here we go."

I looked down and blood was flowing. I was relieved. I didn't want to wait anymore. It was the waiting rooms. If they would have put me back in the room with the bed, it wouldn't have been so bad, but the waiting room with its uncomfortable chairs and overcrowding was not where I wanted to spend another hour or two. Luckily, they had ordered my chemotherapy drugs already, and I was immediately sent to my room.

When I was finally hooked up to an IV at the infusion center, this time I was handed a little cup with three small pills in it as the steroid started to flow.

"What's this?" I asked.

"Zofran."

"Why is it not in IV form?"

A small shrug from the nurse. *"Shortages."*

She didn't have to say much more. It was everywhere now. I had tried to put things up on the social media sites hoping that it would take off. But it never did, only getting reposted by a few others who were fighting cancer themselves. What I couldn't get people to understand and neither could the media was that this was turning into a major problem. Although I personally was focused on cancer drugs, it was also other types of drugs. The lack of safe production in the United States and the dependence on other countries and their facilities was taking a toll on everyone. Drug prices were up exponentially with no end in sight. People who needed life-saving drugs were not getting them–forcing some hospitals to turn to the black market in an effort to save lives. I had been told that even things like steroids were now on the shortage list, saving them for cancer patients and not giving them to orthopedic patients. I thought how wrong that was. We had the technology to replace someone's knee and have them live a life where they could run and walk without pain, but we didn't have enough of the medicines, so that after surgery they could take a few steroids to help with the healing and muscle rebuilding. IV Zofran, although not something that saved my life, definitely made my side-effects within the not-wanting-to-kill-myself range. I understood that the IV version would have to be saved for those who couldn't swallow pills.

"So what's the difference?"

"Mostly timing. IV works faster than pills."

I let myself be ok with that statement, as she gave me the pills almost a full hour earlier than usual. I also asked the question because I didn't want my time spent hooked to an IV shortened because I was so late getting back into my room because of the sheath issue.

Charlotte worked within the hospital system that my cancer hospital was in and always tried to come have lunch with me on infusion days. It gave Sue a chance to get up and stretch her legs and walk around for a little bit. When she arrived, I asked her questions about the difference between the IV Zofran and pill form. Charlotte wasn't a nurse specializing in cancer care but spent years as an ICU nurse then traveled the country as a consultant, and finally decided to come home to stay after her child was born and to work in case management. I knew she had seen a lot and was a wealth of information. She was also intelligent enough when she didn't know something to say so. I liked asking her things because she looked at things not just in my best interest but from the viewpoint of the nurses. If she didn't know something she could point me in the right direction on how to get an answer or what to ask about. She confirmed what the nurse had said about the timing. She was also there when I asked if I could get an antibiotic for a cold that I knew had turned into a sinus infection. My infusion nurse said she would call the nurse practitioner since the doctor was not in on that day. The N.P. refused my request stating the overuse of antibiotics. I was irritated and Charlotte told me to burn up her phone until she gave it to me.

I hated making phone calls and told Charlotte that when I get too sick to do these things myself, she was in charge of making all my calls, and she agreed. This was the kind of information I could get out of Charlotte. I would have let the issue alone after being told no. She let me know I had the right to an antibiotic if I wanted one, and if she wouldn't do it, then call the doctor.

They started the Taxotere drip, and I found out instead of ninety minutes like the Taxol, it would only take an hour. Again, I questioned why and was told that all chemo meds and the amount ordered take different times to administer. It seemed like less medicine to me, then

I remembered the twenty-five percent less statement made by the doctor when telling the oncology nurse what to order. I also wasn't given the Benadryl on this round which was the drug given to me for side-effects that produced its own side-effects! I didn't miss it, and I didn't really care why they had stopped giving it to me.

Even with the extended wait for the medicine to work on the sheath, I left the hospital at the same time as usual. No Zofran drip, no Benadryl, and a shortened time on the Taxotere from the Taxol made up the difference.

The next day, I awoke to a full blown sinus infection and thought I would walk down and see either the doctor or nurse practitioner to show them the yellow goo coming from my nose right after I got my white blood cell raising shot.

At 4pm, I checked in at the lab for my shot and sat down. This was usually a very quick process. There were only a dozen people sitting in the waiting room, not the usual overflow of people. It was twenty minutes before a nurse came out to tell me it would only be a few more minutes and apologized for the delay. I sat there texting whoever I could think of to pass the time. At an hour an ten minutes, another nurse came out again to say she was sorry for the delay.

"What's the problem?"

I was expecting to hear about some type of emergency instead I got:

"We can't find your file for some reason."

"Are you kidding me?!"

I was pissed, and I wasn't about to be left sitting here for hours while in a huge hospital they looked for a file.

"How is that my problem, and how long are you gonna have me sit here?! I've already been here over an hour for something that should have taken ten minutes; you have about twenty minutes left 'til I start vomiting!"

Now the vomiting part was an exaggeration. I actually had about two days before I got to that point, but I wanted to light a fire under everyone within earshot.

"Oh," she paused for a moment. *"You know what, come on back. I'll figure this out."*

I followed her back while she apologized over and over and

started to explain their files. I didn't really care about their paper files versus digital files. I knew what happened. Somebody shoved my file inside someone else's accidentally, and until that other person's file is opened again, nobody will find mine. How do I know that? Because I spent about four months filing in a doctor's office for a friend who needed some extra help. I knew how the color coding worked, and I was warned when I started to be careful not to push the file into its spot too quickly or that would happen. It seemed the most logical thing in my head.

She gave me the shot and said she would keep looking for my file. I was good with that.

CHAPTER THIRTY-FOUR

EVER WONDER WHAT IT'S LIKE TO START DYING?

When my remission ended in August of 2011, I read all the doom and gloom. The facts were staring me in the face. If I couldn't hit another remission, I had 12-18 months. The only evidence to support many of those numbers is when most people give up on their treatment or the treatment gets the better of them.

I paused now in the first days of March of 2012, under technical terms; maybe I have five months left.

With each chemotherapy treatment, the side effects get stronger and hurt more. The body having been worn down from previous treatments doesn't have the ability to 'fight the good fight' as they coin in the cancer world. The slogans start to irritate you when you see them on TV or the internet. The other day, as well-meaning people prepared for the May and June Relay for Life walks, I heard on TV a catch line for those walks:

"When we walk together we are bigger than Cancer."

The only thing I could think of when I heard it is....

Unbelievable! I don't think so! Because we don't walk together. We walk at hundreds of little events, and it's breast cancer against the rest of the cancers vying for the same dollars.

Oh, I know. These types of events are important. For remembering, for raising awareness, for providing money to help; it's a network and a support system for those who need it most.

But like the rest of what I write, let me tell you what the sentence doesn't do.

It doesn't tell you what it is like to *die* from the cancer treatment.

There will be people out there always who will raise their fist to the heavens, like Scarlet O'Hara in Gone With The Wind claiming she will never go hungry again.... and yet, we know... we know with each time we crawl into the bathroom, sitting on the toilet puking into a bucket, that this is not how one should live.

When did I first know I was dying? March 5, 2012. Chemotherapy had been administered seven days earlier. I had heard the doctor when he switched the Taxol to Taxotere to cut the amount by twenty-five percent. Even when it ran in the IV bag, it was two-thirds of the time.

Finishing my Zofran on Sunday afternoon, six days after chemo meant the worst of it was coming. I knew that. My bowels would start to move again after Zofran stops. More intense nausea kicks in, stomach cramping, headache, sweats. I want to say it's like having the stomach flu along with food poisoning. This time add to my mess: a sinus infection that the nurse practitioner refused to give me antibiotics for, a weakened sinus cavity from the Avistin, and a CT scan, that once I got home from the doctor's office almost three weeks ago now showed atrophy of the left kidney and sigma colon. This was a recipe for disaster. Everyone at the cancer center knew all these details, and yet nobody said a word except...

"Your constipation should be better with Taxotere."

Bullshit.

I picked up the Little One from driver's training, a mere five minutes from the house. All day long I knew the explosion was coming, the constant diarrhea with some vomiting until the seven day build-up of toxins, caused by the inability to poop, laxatives and medications that caused constipation was gone from my body. My stomach had been unrelenting in its reminder that grief was on the way. The only relief I had was a reclining position on the couch, from which in true 'Kim' spirit I managed to get in a full six hours of work in. It was the only thing that kept my mind off my increasing discomfort.

I barely made it back into the house from picking up the kids and my stomach was churning. The Little One having been picked up by his grandmother after school of course was 'starving' as was My Other who called to say he was on the way home. I threw pork chops in the oven and went into the bathroom.

The vomiting with severe pain and a week's worth of blood

from my wasted nasal cavities from the former doses of Avastin compounded with the sinus infection drainage started coming up, and my bowels started to move. I thought I would have been spared since the day before I was lucky (if you could call it that) enough to pass two fairly large, rock hard pieces of shit. It was an all-day event to get them out, but I was feeling more confident that this would be easier this time.

Only it didn't stop coming out of me like I had hoped....

For fifty minutes I sat there, stomach cramping, fluids coming out of me, including a nose bleed complete with the sinus infection mucus. I flushed and dumped the bucket over and over. I eventually had to strip off most of my clothing because it was too hard to get up and turn around to dump the bucket with jeans around my ankles. My stomach cramped, my back hurt, and my throat burned. I started crying after about ten minutes of this.

My poor stepson was sitting down the hall doing his homework; I prayed that for once he didn't listen, and he put on his headphones. I was embarrassed and heartbroken that he had to listen to me. The funny thing is, after it was over I snuck into my bedroom half-dressed to put on some pajamas and walked down the hall to where he sat at the dining room table. I longed for our old house where he would have sat upstairs away from all this, quiet and secluded....

"I'm so sorry you had to listen to all that kiddo," I said trying to sound upbeat and normal.

"Huh?" he removed his headphones, and I felt relief.

"I'm sorry you had to listen to all that.... Will you take the pork-chops out of the oven when the timer goes off?"

"It actually just sounds like coughing," he said with a smile... He's such a good kid. I know if the roles were reversed, and I was the kid, I'd be hiding at a friend's house.

I made it back down the hall in time for the whole processes to start over again for another twenty minutes. I could only think how enjoyable The Little One and The Other's dinner was as they had to listen to me vomit while they ate.

After the second round, I got up and saw blood. That is when the fear set in again. You see, as I was throwing up, and saw the pink colored vomit, I had an excuse. My sinuses had been bleeding and you know how that works, when your sinuses are running, no matter how much you blow, some of it you are going to swallow.

Now I needed to know–was I peeing this blood and having a kidney problem? Or was it a bowel problem? I knew the differences between bright red and black blood and what they meant. What I had going for me was this was bright red, but there were a couple ounces of it… Something had come apart within me, I thought for sure.

During the last chemo round, I had had some of the bright red blood at the end of a similar but shorter episode and it had stopped not long after it started. I had dismissed it as a hemorrhoid.

I cleaned myself up again and went to lie on the bed. My stomach and bowels were still churning. Everything within me had felt wrong. I laid there and cried, knowing that this is what I had to look forward to for the next few months, and wondering if I would be able to take much more. I tried to calm myself down, as did Chris.

I had already resorted to my new 'pass-out' position in bed: sitting upright and sideways, crouched in the fetal position trying to get the internal pains to go away.

I tried desperately to relax; only my mind couldn't help but think about all I had been through in the past two hours…

Is this going to get worse?

Can I handle more than this?

Is this why they morphine-up people?

I was too literal of a thinker; I kept going back to Betty Eadie's words from her books. About how wonderful and loving Jesus and God were, how she longed to be back with them. I tried desperately to take comfort in that and my Catholic upbringing of a wonderful heaven; yet I was terrified to leave this existence and leave Chris and Hunter…

I worried endlessly about both of them and who would be there for them in the role that I played. Hunter always had his mom to turn to, but Chris and I had formed this bond of togetherness. I knew in eternity we would be together, but another forty years of him being here by himself tore at my very soul. As I lay there knowing my days were quickly coming to an end, the emotional hurt that I was going to inflict on Chris was tearing at me at an even greater rate than the physicality's were, I was now fighting on two fronts...

Physical and Emotional...

And my power was weakening; I was convinced that I had started the process of death.

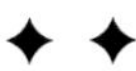

The hardest thing? Nothing stops for you. It all keeps moving forward.

Because I had gotten so incredibly sick this last round, I knew I still had to deal with the effects of the Neulasta at the ten day mark. I sat in bed the next day, worrying, crying. It was Tuesday, exactly a week since the infusion. I was deathly sick and couldn't get myself to do anything except lay there going in and out of sleep. Chris had taken Wednesday, Thursday and Friday off because he knew The Little One had a lot going on that week. Between driving lessons and school, he knew I was never that great a week after chemo. His being home those days got me out of bed and moving around. He even got me to go to the store a couple of times, although the visits were short.

My uncle passed away, losing his own cancer battle, and the funeral was that week. My uncle had been at my wedding eleven months earlier. Although he was up there in years on God's Earth, it was still a hard hit knowing he was taken from us via this horrible thing.

With all this going on in my life, I still never felt the rebound like I usually do of feeling a little better every day. I forgot about the shot of Neulasta and the second wave of vomiting that usually hit me when it didn't come on day ten. In my quest to forget about the round of terror and the thought of dying, I had gone ahead and I made plans against Chris's better judgment to go visit with Brian and Danielle on Saturday.

Friday night after dinner (which consisted of nothing more than a leftover baked potato) the pains in my stomach started, like someone stabbing me with a knife while I had horrible gas pains.

Chris played his guitar next to me to try and soothe me and help me fall asleep. It worked, and although I woke up with the nausea and no pains, again by the time lunch rolled around on Saturday, the pain had returned. By 4pm, I was sound asleep in bed. I set my alarm knowing we had made plans for 6:40pm, knowing I could get up and go if I got the chance to rest. I did just that, taking ginger ale and saltines with me.

"Do you have enough stuff?" The Other asked as we were walking out seeing the nearly empty two liter in my hand with a half a sleeve of saltines.

"It's Danielle. She'll have stuff for me."

Danielle was always prepared. As the couple hosted parties and events over the years, and we visited on a regular basis, no matter what came up—Danielle was always prepared. I wasn't wrong this time either. She had a full box of crackers and a few cans of ginger ale.

Part of the fun at our friend's house was the food; we would sit at the kitchen table, laugh and talk while Brian kept bringing out snacks. Chris and I don't keep a lot of things like that in our house because they simply aren't in the grocery budget, so it was always a treat to go there and snack. I knew I wouldn't be able to snack on that night, and I thought the saltines and ginger ale would help settle my stomach. The longer we sat there the more the smells started bother me. Brian noticed it.

"Does all this stuff bother you?"

Not wanting to wreck everyone else's fun, I sucked it up and said no. I made it about ninety minutes before I knew it was time to go.

We got home and I went to bed. Stomach pains back and nausea getting worse, I lay there for hours. Finally at 4 am, it started. I went to the bathroom and the water and ginger ale I had been sipping because of dry mouth came up. I couldn't believe that almost two weeks later, I was still getting sick. I thought about how ridiculous this all was. *I wouldn't have any time to do anything,* I kept thinking. *I can't be sick for two weeks. There is no recovery time.* I prayed for a remission. I needed a break, a few months like before so I could rebuild a little. I felt like the more of these hour-long vomiting sessions I had, the harder it was to recover from them.

I knew then that if I didn't hit a remission, the treatment—not the cancer—was going to kill me.

✦ ✦

I continued to get sick over and over for several hours. When it finally stopped, I was bed-ridden for the rest of Sunday and through the night. Chris kept encouraging me to try and take small bites of food and to drink as much water as I could. I got a couple of glasses of water down and a couple of glasses of lemon-lime soda. Food was very limited. I ate one yogurt, one bite of a brownie, and a few saltines throughout the day. It wasn't much, but it was something. I managed to do all of it from a reclined position as I still couldn't sit upright.

I was never a great sleeper. I used to, in my early twenties stay up partying until three or four in the morning and then getting up at seven to be to work at 8am. I can still remember the feeling of the alarm going off and the shakiness from the previous night's alcohol still in my veins. Yet, once I was up and moving, I was fine. I never really got much more than four hours a night my whole life; oh, I would go to bed but lay there for hours thinking, dreaming, and planning my life. I loved the quiet of my room at those moments. It wasn't until I was diagnosed with cancer and in treatment when I decided to actually get up when I wasn't sleeping; there was nothing left to dream and plan for. I felt it a waste of the precious moments I had left on this earth to lie there and worry about what was to come, not to mention that the dream of the future was over. I entertained myself writing, watching TV and reading; quiet activities that wouldn't upset the sleep of the rest of the house.

Yet, there were days like today. After the ravaging side-effects, I wanted nothing more than to sleep. No dreams just to be able to rebuild and recoup. The last time I remember having fallen asleep was for a few hours on Sunday morning. I was still feeling sick to my stomach, and I had been counting the minutes until something would come on TV that would take my mind off my own illness. I had put my head down and I know I had slept for about ninety minutes. Before that, it would have been Friday night, when I actually got a solid five or six hours. So with days with no sleep, confounded by the ravaging side-effects, I wanted nothing more than to rest. Yet, sleep eluded me, as usual.

I sipped my warm ginger ale, wishing I had the strength to go and get more ice. I felt hungry but had no energy to get out of bed and make myself something.

Food is a huge issue with chemotherapy. I was told originally you have to eat what your body craves. It's easier on the stomach, I was craving scrambled eggs. But I knew I couldn't wake Chris to make them, he had to work tomorrow, and I couldn't do it. So I sat there stomach aching still from the vomiting and hungry to boot.

To amuse myself, I would go on cancer sites and read their side-effects list neatly laid out in black and white. I found one that listed the percentage you have to vomit from your chemotherapy drugs, and was not surprised to read that ninety percent of the people taking my two drugs vomit. No shit.

I guess it's the way these sites make their lists, like they are no big deal. *"Take care of yourself, and everything will be okay."*

Yeah, right.

I thought about the severe battle I had just encountered with the never-ending side-effects and what would happen if I taped it? Would it go viral? People loved all this gross horror at the movies and on TV–what if I brought them real horror? Would it spur someone or maybe no one into action? There have been shows and movies dealing with the subject of cancer, yet they focused on the emotional connections more than the physical side-effects. What if I took that emotional connection away and showed the nitty-gritty of it? The biggest dilemma is how to cover my lower half during the filming, maybe a makeshift half wall, where you would see where I was sitting, but couldn't see the actual working parts on me; I wanted people to hear it, to realize how you have to cope with this killer.

Vomit is a funny sketch on adult cartoons; I've laughed myself numerous times at these types of things, but the sheer complexity of having to take care of yourself while this is going on is difficult. Would I like someone there to grab the bucket and replace it with a fresh smelling clean one? Of course I would. But who in their right mind would do such a thing, and where are they going to dump the used bucket?

Then, I came up with what I needed, two toilets facing each other…

If I had only known years ago, I would have designed a house like that…

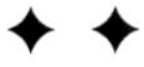

Monday morning, I dragged myself out of bed and drove the Little One to school. It was going to be a busy week again and this time I didn't have Chris to help me. I prayed that I would get better as the week progressed. I came home and sat on the couch in an upright position for over ninety minutes and then got up to make myself a little something to eat. It was exhausting to stand in the kitchen for a few minutes, but as usual, I pushed myself. I ate something small and decided to take a shower. I peed right before the shower and noticed a foul smell and thought, 'I really need a shower.' I showered and got dressed.

The water from the shower burned my numb toes but to accommodate my toes the water would be too cold for the rest of me. Always in the habit of using one of those ultra-scented body washes, I poured it on until it was all I could smell. I had been told by several people that their side-effects include the inability to use any product with a scent or other chemicals, I felt happy that I could still use all my personal care products. I exited the shower and dried off. It was strange because I thought I had to pee again. I sat down and did, even though it was only a minor amount. I dressed and straighten up the bathroom and again thought I had to pee.

I went to the other bathroom in the house because I kept the scale in the half bath. I wanted to weigh myself to see if the bloating was happening with me that I had read about with the Taxotere. When I sat down to pee, the smell was back. I smelled worse than the outhouse-again! I felt like I had to pee and couldn't.

The first thing that came to mind was some type of infection or a problem with the stent. I knew from the last CT-Scan that my left kidney and sigma colon were atrophied according to the radiologist; the doctor made no real mention of it during our visit, so I tried not to worry. The websites said that Taxol can cause neuropathy not only of the hands and feet but colon also. This new smell… was this stuff that has been inside of me for days, is that why? Were things starting to move again? I had an appointment with the urologist already scheduled next week. I crossed my fingers and hoped for the best and that maybe the issue was because the stent needed to be replaced.

Until then, we had a new side-effect added to the crop: the constant, ever-present, never-ending need to pee—complete with gagging smell!

The smell issues with the pee stopped after a day, and a few days later, as was the pattern, my poop started coming out, in what had become normal for me, only it also was accompanied by a smell. A chemical type smell, like nail polish remover; I couldn't believe things could get more disgusting than they already had been.

That smell also subsided after a few days and a new side-effect reared its nasty head. I had lost the ability to taste. My dad had said a few months into his treatment, as my mom complained about all the food he was wasting, *"Everything just tastes eh."*

As my taste buds became damaged, the big eater that I was started to vanish. Everything tasted exactly the same… like nothing… it is the weirdest feeling. It is like eating when everything tastes like spit. Yep that's right. Think about the saliva in your mouth. Kind of gross huh? Imagine if no matter what you ate, the textures would be different, but it all tastes the same. Water was the worst. It was like drinking down large quantities of spit. I would try to make the water as cold as possible because I could tell the difference between temperatures. This way the cold feeling would make things less gross. It was hard to explain to people but they would bring me water with two or three ice cubes in it and that would frustrate me.

My whole life I liked cold drinks, but it was now crucial for me to get the water down. And, it was like I was constantly begging for someone to bring me more ice to put in my water.

I now knew what my dad meant. I would open the refrigerator or cupboard and see something and my brain would say that sounds good–knowing what the taste would be. However, when I ate it, the taste I was expecting didn't happen. I tried many, many things, and quickly learned to make myself only a bite or two. Because if I couldn't get it down with just the texture of the product, I wasn't going to eat it. Luckily, after four days, it went away, and my taste buds would return to almost 'normal.'

The third week in March, I headed out to see the Urologist. It was a simple visit; pee in a cup, take some vitals and the doctor was in to see me. The stent was going on seven months old and had to be swapped out. There was no more waiting. They would call me with the surgery date. Again, they weren't doing it in the outpatient center but in the actual hospital…just in case.

I hate that just in case.

I got the call from the office two days later. They scheduled me eight days after chemo. I argued and said I needed at least twelve. No go. I went to see my oncologist for the usual pre-chemo visit, and he agreed that I needed ten to twelve days. I dropped the ball and didn't insist on a reschedule–fueled by that part of me that hates making phone calls.

When I woke up on the morning of my doctor's visit pre-chemo, I knew I had some great things working in my favor. My last doctor's visit, my CA125 was eighty-two and then I had a chemo. I was hoping that when I went for my labs this morning it was going to be great news. I might only need this one more or perhaps this one and the one after it; I was excited driving downtown. I had my little talk with the Almighty like I always did. I was smart enough to grab a half a sandwich, bottle of water and granola bar. The last time I had sat for hours waiting for the doctor on an empty stomach.

I looked around as I drove. We had experienced a great two weeks of beautiful summer weather, very unusual for Michigan in

Mid-March. The trees were flowering, daffodils and crocuses along with pansies were blooming everywhere. I loved flowers and enjoyed all the color that was reflecting in the sun. The temperature had dropped almost forty degrees from the eighty degrees we had been experiencing, but it was still magnificent out.

I always loved the seasons in Michigan. Their beauty and how a sunny day could bring out the best in people. Some years, our winters could be so long they would drag from month to month, and it reflected in everyone's attitude. This early break made it so much nicer.

As I approached the downtown area, people were out in force on this sunny morning. Walking back and forth from their cars to jobs or school; the city was having its issues, but there were still some who believed in it and were trying desperately to have it make a real comeback as a destination city.

As I admired everything in my path, I hoped that I wasn't setting myself up for disappointment. I tried after the change to the new cancer center not to think about an end date, the next remission. I mentioned it to close friends and family after the eighty-two number came up but until this morning I hadn't really hoped and prayed. I started to worry myself. What if the new chemo didn't work? What if my number went up? What if I needed four more? I went from being content to upset. When they took my vitals, my heart rate and blood pressure was up. Some call that the 'white coat' syndrome—Nervous to see the doctor. I was never nervous to see the doctor. It was the waiting that irritated me. My last visit here was hours. This time I was already working on forty-five minutes with no one having been called back yet. I knew once they called me, I was still a minimum of thirty minutes from seeing the doctor. Someone in the waiting room was obviously having some type of bowel distress because the small waiting room smelled horrible, and, as they had more and more people enter the clinic area, it seemed to make it worse.

I had been waiting now on doctors and for treatments for going on two years. I never have gotten used to it. I understand the concept. Emergencies come up, people are fit in, and mostly–I don't want to be rushed when speaking to my doctor, and I would expect him to sit and talk to all his patients. That takes time. It is something you have to get your head around and accept. What I can't figure out is why hospitals don't allow their doctors to book patients at one every fifteen minutes instead of the usual three in every fifteen minute slot. Oh yeah, like I said, I helped out a friend for a few months in a doctor's office. On Saturdays, the girls booked four every fifteen minutes because they were only open from 8 am to 12 pm. The waiting room was a zoo. Angry people were everywhere. When I asked about the policy, they shrugged. The average time in that office was ten minutes with a patient. Cancer patients and their families have a lot of questions. They need guidance and want answers. Spread the appointments out farther apart, or at least call and say,

"We are running an hour behind. Can you come a little later?"

Of course I can! I would rather sit at home or work than sit in the chair at the clinic for more than an hour. It makes sense. The hours are extended by the sheer fact of the number of patients being allowed through the door. Instead the answer to the problem by hospital administrators is to tell the doctors to 'go faster' 'spend less time with each patient.' Really? In a situation where death is the eventual outcome you want to run people through like a drive-thru window at McDonalds? McDonalds is the best, I see the sign on their wall next to the drive-thru window. "GOAL: 30 second DRIVE-THRU." I like that. It's why, when given a choice, I pick their drive-thru over the competition. With that said, it is not the way I select my doctor to treat my cancer! I want, as do most people, a doctor who isn't rushed, who takes the time to explain and answer questions. So why can't the administrators see that as a good thing? Oh right… money… doctors who talk to their patients and spend more than three minutes with them don't bring in as much.

When I finally got to see the doctor, he walked in with a few papers in his hand and no information at his disposal that I needed to see. He joked,

"Your file is getting smaller."

"Is that a good thing?" I joked back.

"No." He looked at the aide and the resident. *"Have we found it yet?"*

"No." They said quietly.

"You aren't switching to another hospital are you?"

"No. They couldn't find my file when I came for my shot after chemo either."

He turned and looked at the aide and in an I-mean-business-voice he said, *"Find her file."* The aide left the room.

He reviewed my treatment, and I immediately asked about remission since the number was eighty-two last time.

"We'll talk when you are under ten."

"I thought it was under thirty-five?"

"We'll look at it again when it's under ten."

"Like less often or less chemo?"

"We'll talk about it then."

My heart sank. I wasn't stupid, and as I drove home I thought about the long conversation of examples he had with me. Why it was important with ovarian cancer to make sure that number was under ten. It was exactly what happened at the other hospital, the number went down with the last treatment to twenty-six, the next month to sixteen, then a month later to twenty-four. I remember asking about it, and was fed that song and dance about it can go up and down under thirty-five. Nope this doctor was right; it kept going up. Only they didn't check me monthly, instead, they moved it to three months, and by that time I was way out of control.

I had to qualify what he said. Re-evaluate under ten. Okay. I had forgotten to get about the new number. I was going to need four more to get me under ten, then what? I knew what he was saying and I didn't have to ask. I recalled what the nurse said on my first visit.

"He will never take you off chemo. You will have to tell him when you are done."

I was going to be like my dad, on chemo until something else got me. I knew I had to do something to organically help my chances of keeping my body in as best shape possible to help me withstand the years that I had watched my dad go through.

Now I was stuck in the same trap.

Receiving chemotherapy until my last breath, or until I couldn't stand the side-effects anymore.

Terminal cancers were nothing to mess with. One wrong move

and you are done. The choice to move to this cancer hospital I figured, even though I was disappointed, more than likely bought me another couple of years.

I got home and took a look in the mirror: my jowls had dropped; my skin was wrinkling; I had aged in this last round to look my full forty-nine years. I had turned into a middle-aged woman in less than a year, and I needed to do something about that also. On Danielle's 30th birthday, she announced that she was irritated because I was ten years older and looked younger than her. Of course I never thought that. It's nice to know she did. People were always mistaking me for a few years younger than I actually was.

Now cancer was taking that away from me.

I went back to the books from the people who had survived cancer and read more about what they did with diet and exercise to help themselves.

As I headed with Danielle to chemo number eight, not making the call to change my surgery was on my mind, but I had a new attitude... For the hundredth time... I wanted to treat this round differently. No more laxatives and stool softeners. I made a shopping list by going online and trying to figure out every high fiber food I could eat without chemicals. I was thinking about all of this when I went back to get my IV started.

The nurse pulled a couple vials of blood with no problem, and then it slowed down drastically. It took a long time by her hand-suctioning the blood to pull it out before she got enough to fill the rest of the long skinny tubes. When I returned to the waiting room hallway, Danielle was standing. She had given up her seat to a cancer patient because, as usual, they were out of seats. As it was, we were in the hallway and not the main room. Again people were sitting on the floor waiting.

"Wow you were back there a long time," she stated.

So, it wasn't just me thinking it took forever; I explained to her what happened. Danielle knew what a sheath was which was good;

I figured she wouldn't be surprised if I got stuck here on one of our trips for the extra hour if they had to insert the medicine again, which, judging by the slow draw, was coming again. I thought, *well, at least I am learning as I go at this center.*

I was surprised but not shocked when they took me to a chair and not a bed this time. Judging by the actual time lapse to administer the complete infusion, I really didn't need a bed even though I liked it. The chairs were the same as the first hospital; only instead of one private room, there were many semi-private rooms with brick walls in-between chairs and curtains at the front. There were still two additional chairs, so Danielle could sit and set our stuff on the other one.

This time at the start, I was handed five little blue pills in a cup.

"What's this?"

"Your Decadron."

Steroids are given for various reasons during chemotherapy; to help with nausea, to prevent tumor growth and in some instances to prevent cancer cells from reproducing. She hung the Zofran, and I was pleased with the switch. If I had to choose between the two, in pill form, it would be the steroid. The day progressed without incident, and we headed for home two hours earlier than usual.

CHAPTER THIRTY-FIVE
TRYING AGAIN

Feeling pretty good, I sat down to plan my strategy for food and exercise once again. Armed with the recent revelation that I was stuck in this downward spiral, I wanted to make whatever time I had left manageable and at a quality I could live with. I knew I didn't want to turn into one of those people I saw at the cancer center, clinging to life in a way that required constant assistance. I had spent a full day researching different natural ways to stop or prevent constipation. I had my water up to three quarts a day going into chemo, and although water made me sick while on chemo, I vowed that, no matter what, I would keep drinking it. Every site promoted water as a way to keep things moving. I had also stocked up on and made individual containers with cooked vegetables. I cooked the old standby that I ate while in remission for months.

Broccoli
Cauliflower
Mushrooms
Green Beans
Asparagus
Tomatoes

Armed with a dozen small plastic containers of the mixture, and chopped lettuce as well as salad toppings I liked, and a full batch of Jenn's vegetarian soup. I was ready.

Every day I let Chris drive Hunter to school, so I could sleep for as long as I felt I needed. Then, I would get up, force myself to drink at least ten ounces of water and eat some watermelon, oranges or apples that I had also pre-cut. I would then head for the treadmill and walk for ten minutes. Every two hours, I would eat one of the vegetable mixtures tossed with red wine vinegar and olive oil along with spices like turmeric, black pepper and garlic, along with a full glass of water. Every day, I also tried to drink a ten ounce glass of apple cider or cranberry juice. I kept at it, when I couldn't walk on the treadmill I moved to the stationery sit-down bike Michaelene had loaned me. I drank no pop, but I did add a little of that powder lemonade or ice tea mix to the water about twice a day, making sure I only used half the amount just to give me some taste. By Saturday, I had pooped every day; not a lot, just a very small, hard amount, but it was better than nothing. I tried not to take as many Ativans, saving them only for the worst three nights and cutting the pill in half. I also, because of the upcoming surgery for the stent, wasn't allowed to take the Motrin. My legs hurt and twitched, but I used the Ativan at those times to try and sleep through it. By the weekend, I was moving a lot less and not drinking the required amount of water. My consumption of the veggies had stopped—replaced by small amounts of carbs like noodles and crackers. I had also had a small glass or two of pop. I was irritated with myself yet pleased that I made it five days. On Sunday and Monday, I felt bad. I thought the vomiting was going to start and even tried to force it to start to get it over with. I was panicking about the surgery now. If by eating like this, I had delayed my getting sick, there was no way I could go into surgery vomiting. I had convinced myself I needed to cancel. Chris on the other hand wasn't pleased with this decision. We talked on and off about it; he tried to tell me this was all the usual stuff, and I said no, it wasn't. I was going to be sick during surgery.

I woke up Tuesday, eight days after the chemo infusion, still having not gotten sick or had a decent crap. I didn't feel as horrible as I usually do at eight day mark, so I went to the hospital. Once there, I told every person I came in contact with.... I'm eight days out of chemo and I don't want to get sick. I have a history of vomiting. The anesthesiologist said she would *"hook me up with some good anti-nausea drugs."* I was pleased with that.

The nurse who started my IV for the surgery was training another nurse. She tied the tourniquet and started to talk. I was irritated at the length of time she left it on my arm but listened as she explained how to place the IV between ventricles and why certain size needles were used for catheters to pump the IV medicines. It was a learning experience for me. I knew this new nurse wanted to put the IV in my arm I interjected before she had a chance to ask:

"You'll have to try inserting on a newbie. I'm going through chemotherapy and I know when I've been poked correctly, and I will tell you to get lost if you are fishing around for a vein."

"It's funny you would say that cause the other nurse had a hard time getting a vein on that patient and had to call for help."

The patient in the next curtained waiting area in pre-op was giving everyone a run for their money. She had pulled out her IV twice while I was laying there and refused to do other things and answer questions. The nurse taking care of her looked disheveled and tired from dealing with her. She had gotten the full attention of several of the staff and was being administered to at the expense of others.

The doctor stopped by to check on me before the surgery; I was hoping that he wasn't going to tell me I was second in line. He smiled at me and patted my shin like last time,

"How are you feeling today Kim?"

I knew this doctor had a good sense of humor because of how he tried to joke with The Other instead of panicking, like previous people had done, so I quipped back:

"No... how are you doing? You are the one who has to work today! I'm the one that gets to lay here and enjoy a good nap!"

He laughed at my comment and said, *"Ok, we'll see you in a few minutes."* Meaning I was first.

I went into surgery and came out with the only issue of having to pee like the last time. I asked for Chris, and they said they couldn't find him and that he had stepped out. I knew Chris well enough to know that he had stepped nowhere. Sure enough, when they got sick of me asking for him every time a person walked by my curtained post-op spot, they finally 'found him' sitting in a chair right in front of the reception desk. The volunteer who brought him back took him into the wrong curtained post-op area. I could see him looking around on the other side of the room. I finally got his attention, and he walked over. He was irritated when he found out I had been out of surgery for over forty-five minutes. However, with our experience at that hospital, it really wasn't unexpected.

"What's all the commotion?" he said, motioning to the curtained space next to me.

Once again the patient on the other side of the curtain was commanding the attention of several nurses. They thought she had lost consciousness. I could hear them talking about how her vitals were fine. I could hear what sounded like snoring coming from the room as they kept yelling her name and trying to wake her. Doctors were called, and finally her son showed up. She was sleeping. He told the nurses she always falls into a deep sleep, and you can't wake her up.

"Been doin' it since I was a little kid." I heard what sounded like an older gentleman say.

I thought to myself, you or your mom didn't think that that was important to note with the medical staff? Because of that incident, I stayed in post-op pretty much unattended. I was up when they wheeled me in, asked a few questions, checked some vitals and asked if I wanted graham crackers and juice. I said yes, and they left me two juices and graham crackers, and because of the woman next to me, I didn't see a nurse again until Chris walked in. When she poked her head in again and asked if I wanted to sit in a chair.

"Yes I do, and I need to pee."

"It's just from the surgery."

"Yeah, that's what they said last time I had this surgery, and I peed…a lot." I said to the wall because she didn't listen.

Another hour passed and a second nurse came in and said that she was back from lunch to the girls in the nurse's station, and she headed towards me.

"How do you feel? Ready to go home?"

Oh, so that was the issue! My attending nurse was at lunch. Now I remember why I left this facility!

"Yeah, and I need to pee."

"I'm sure you do. You've had a bag of saline and two juices. I'll have the aide take you soon as you're dressed."

Then she explained the discharge rules to Chris, and she had him sign the paperwork she had explained. I dressed and within minutes the aide was there. I peed for what seemed like an eternity and afterward the feeling that I needed to go never went away. *Ever.* Two weeks after the surgery and I still felt like I always had to go, especially if I stood a lot, walked around or exercised. That could put a crimp in what I wanted to start doing in the quest to try and better my quality of life.

I pushed through the feeling and tried not to think about it as much as possible. I knew I would have actually traded the having to pee every hour over this. At least, then I actually went and felt relief afterwards. *Going pee and then never feeling satisfied afterwards sucks.*

I felt good all day following the surgery. I figured it was all the anti-nausea meds they gave me, and I knew one of them was Zofran because I couldn't poop for the next two days. By the weekend, I felt decent. I had continued on the diet high in fruits, vegetables, water, and green tea. Saving soft drinks for specialties like eating in a restaurant. I also continued to walk on the treadmill daily and use the stationary bike. Not every day was perfect, but I thought that in doing this I might be able to start tolerating the treatments better. Although it was no picnic, the start of this process kept me from the explosive vomiting and diarrhea that I had been suffering with. I also made a note of the fact that I did have a second round of anti-nausea meds brought on by the surgery. Which might have helped limit the amount of vomiting; I wasn't above administering a second round of anti-nausea meds on the second week in the future. However, what really stuck in my mind was the fact that for the first time during chemo, I didn't take anything to try and help the constipation. I also didn't take any Motrin and I limited my Ativan use to only three half pills. I was going to try that again along with only eating fruits and vegetables on the first few days along with Jenn's vegetarian soup. Just to see if it might help me.

I knew it wasn't a perfect plan, but it was all I had.

CHAPTER THIRTY-SIX

SOMETIMES YOU JUST HAVE TO VENT

Dear Diary,

Today I feel…

-My head is pounding; not like a headache, just one spot on the top left side.

-My nose aches; not from a cold, but from the lack of nose hairs, which is now causing random small bits of blood to form. It makes the inside of my nose dry and itchy. However you don't want to blow, wipe, itch or generally press on the area for fear of causing a much larger problem.

-My left leg aches. Kind of like growing pains. From my hip all the way down to my toes, it never stops. If I can convince The Other to rub or massage it for any length of time, with any kind of pressure, I can get several moments of relief while the act is being done.

-To go along with it, my knee caps throb.

-The heartburn is unbearable.

-The shooting pains in my stomach are new, but expected.

-The feeling of constantly having to urinate at least offers me the exercise of going back to the bathroom several times an hour.

-The numbness in my hands now includes all but my pinky fingers.

-The numbness in my feet goes to both ankles.

-I have random wounds now appearing; pin size open sores that bleed for a day then seal back up.

-My fingernails feel as if they have been smashed in a door.

-My gums are receding so bad around the only crown I have in my mouth that I rinse and floss after anything that goes in my mouth for fear of having even more issues.

...And this is a GOOD day on chemo.

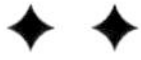

I was doing some research on ovarian cancer, and the more I do, it seems the angrier I get. It wasn't long ago that a famous celebrity was out pitching her movie, and of course, as all reporters do, the digging for any interesting information not related to the movie starts...

Turns out, she is an ovarian cancer survivor; the doctor caught it in Stage I. Seems she spit up some food like a baby would. BAM! To the doctor and a correct diagnosis! Must be nice to be one of the wealthy, with doctors that will take the time to listen to you, run the proper test and not dismiss it as the symptoms of a menopausal woman. With that said, I could be wrong, after all Gilda Radner jumped up and down and screamed... no doctors listen to her.

Yeah, I can see Miss Average at her yearly gynecological visit....

"So, I'm also having these digestive issues. My food keeps coming back up. I spit up like a baby would."

"Take some antacids. You know you're not twenty anymore. You can't eat like you used to. Stay away from spicy foods."

How do I know that? Because the first time that happened to me was in 2004. I *told* the doctor du jour that I was having a hard time getting foods to settle, and that they would come back up. He told me it could be acid reflux, heartburn, try some antacids. Seriously, it is now 2012! I am sitting here with side-effect after side-effect, and we could have done something in 2004? *Diary is disgusted*

Yeah, well, I guess you need a Hollywood doctor for that.

I was amazed as I listened to the online videos of interview after interview with this celeb. She kept all this to herself, even going to treatments alone. To each his own, but herein lays the point I am desperately trying to get out there...

We need to be louder as a nation, as a people, as Human Beings. We need big names and big money behind this cancer or many more including myself are going to die. This disease in all its forms and its treatments are so horrific and so devastating that we hide in a closet, afraid to tell people that–*It hurts to go poop, or worse I can't go poop. I vomit all over myself.* The pain is so unbearable. I want to sit and cry as the people around me tell me, *"You can do it." "Hang in there." "We need you." Or worse yet, "Don't worry, soon this will be over so you can get on with your life".*

Caught you off guard with that last one didn't I Diary? *Diary nods head yes*

Yeah, you see the looks. They want you around, but they want you back the way you were. Funny, happy, the person they call up to make the party a little better. Now they don't know what to say to you or are afraid you will drone on about your issues. They are tired; tired of cleaning up after you, making you food so you can throw it up, massaging where it hurts, and holding your hand while you cry. They want their life partner back, their friend, their sister, and are trying to force you to take or do anything the doctor says in order to send you into a remission that will allow them a couple more 'good' weeks.

Many of my acquaintances left diary, it's hard when you can't sit around and booze every weekend or go out on a moment's notice. *Diary is sad* Oh don't worry my dear confidant, the good ones stayed. They hung in there with me and suffered along side of me. *Diary feels better now*

I found myself at many a crossroad. Wanting to deal with the chemo and its effects and telling the doctor, no more Neulasta, no more Avastin; just shoot me up every four weeks, call it a maintenance drug, and be done with it. However, I read that these things *can* help people add two months to their lives. I am now sitting here half way to life expectancy. Those two months are important; as they would be to any mother, father, wife, husband, sister, brother, son or daughter. Like, maybe I get 14-20 months instead of the 12-18 months originally assigned by the internet doctors.

Yes, Diary, I sit wide awake and in pain from every direction. *"You need to rest. Get some sleep."* Yes, you are correct. I encourage you to review the list of symptoms. Could you sleep? Oh don't worry diary. They give you a supply of aids, in my case Ativan. I could put myself into a drug-induced sleep. The pill works for about two hours, but is this really how I want to spend my last months of life, sleeping on and off with pills in hand?

The list of celebrities that have had or died from ovarian cancer is long, and yet except for the noise made by Gilda Radner about ovarian cancer, nobody comes forward to yell and scream. Ovarian needs to be one of the fashionable cancers. Ever try to find a Teal Ribbon in the store? They are all pink. Breast cancer advocates have done their job, got the word out, and they still have an amazingly long way to go. Ovarian cancer needs to catch up. They say on the websites, *"Pump Up The Volume," "Fight Like A Girl," or "Break The Silence."* These are great slogans and we need to get them out there. *Diary agrees*

I found out in my many discussions with people at the cancer center that the wife of a local celebrity has ovarian cancer. She has been in remission awhile and raises money for the cancer hospital. Good for her, however she never uses her husband's celebrity status to get the word out. Maybe she should?

I guess some people just don't have it in them to get out there and *"Pump Up The Volume" and "Fight Like A Girl."* It is not within them to *"Break The Silence."* Everyone has their own calling in these matters, but I can still be angry about it. That's my right. Am I wrong here Diary?

What's that you say diary? Be the one, the one to *"Fight Like A Girl" and "Pump Up The Volume" then "Break The Silence".*

Hmm.... It's a thought... And you know diary, you are right. I am the one.

No matter how many dinners I wreck for people talking about vomit and my lack of pooping abilities.

I need to speak up. Then, maybe others will also.

Diary agrees

Hey diary, do you think they'll let me talk about this on Morning TV?

"Yes Mrs. Henderly what is your book about?"

"I couldn't take a shit for eight days straight, and when I finally did it came out of both ends"

Think the audience would set down their cereal spoons Diary?

Diary Laughs

CHAPTER THIRTY-SEVEN
GROUPIES HAPPEN

So many things happened as I went through this process. The funniest and weirdest one is groupies.

Groupies are the people who are attracted to the money, the power, or the celebrity status of an individual. They are most often associated with rock-and-roll, but watching the number of politicians and other celebrities that take a tumble, they are heavily vested everywhere.

I was no stranger to them. Having been involved in music, I saw them everywhere and laughed as they vied for The Other's attention as well as his band mates over the years. The wives and girlfriends of these guys used to laugh at the lengths girls would go to talk to a guy playing part-time in a cover band.

However, when they appeared on the social media sites after I got sick, offering to "be there" to "talk" if my husband needed. I was amazed. Never inquiring about me, but "worried about him." How desperate were these women that they would want to hook up with a man whose wife was dying, and what does it say about the man if he chooses to go? My husband ignored the request–seeing through the veiled attempts at his attention. You must know that attention is very addictive and the unaware can be caught off-guard at the attempts to form 'relationships' when a person is hurting. This goes for men and women. There are as many male groupies as there are female.

Of course The Other had a history with these types of women, so his senses were always on guard for self-serving woman looking for a hard-working man to leach onto and drain of assets or become a baby daddy. Having seen first-hand what lengths these types of people will go to.

It has made him skeptical of all attempts at relationships that seem self-serving.

My only advice is to be wary of random people that show up out of nowhere to only help the spouse of someone suffering. It should be noted that this happens at all ages. After my grandfather got sick and elderly gentleman showed up at my grandmother's door 'just to talk'. She sent him packing with a wave of her arm. It made me laugh and proud that my grandmother knew the difference.

"All chemo did for my mom was wear her down. It didn't take away any cancer; if anything, it allowed the cancer to kick her in the ass."

- Haley Dempster
Daughter of my friend Karen Dempster who lost her battle in the cancer war in December 2011.

REGRETS AND THE FINAL CURTAIN

When I think back about the symptoms and how they crept in, I can see why *sans* modern medicine that people died centuries before and that the median age was barely in the fifties. I can't imagine, ending everything now, at the ripe old age of forty-nine. Am I ready? Definitely. Do I want to? Most certainly not. I guess the difference in those two statements is very plain. *If* I would have known that my expiration date was going to be fifty and not seventy or eighty like I originally thought, I probably would have done things a little bit differently in my life.

I would have gone to the doctor when I was sick. If I would have put *me* before money, I would have caught this earlier and had a much better chance at a little more life. The fact that I thought of my jobs and my bosses first, before my own better health is something that I can never really come to terms with. It is sad, because in the long run, not one of my former bosses ever put me before their bottom line.

> I would have not have had an unyielding pursuit of fabulous credit and good banking habits. I would have lived more like the general public. Borrow, borrow, borrow and who cares.
>
> I would have eliminated people from my life that were a drain a lot faster than I did.
>
> I would have never worked a holiday or a Sunday; instead I would have spent that time with my family.
>
> I would have told someone from my past to his face that he was a brilliant man and that I learned a lot from him. That's hard for someone like me who already thought she knew everything. In the same breath, I would have told him that he was a complete jackass, and that the way he treats people only shows what an insecure small-minded person he really is.
>
> I would have trusted my gut more and went with the status quo less.

I would have gone to school to be a teacher or a social worker.

I would have made myself more technologically adept.

I would have eaten more fruits and vegetables and less sugar.

I would have paid attention to the second-hand smoke I was inhaling and the chemicals I was putting in my body.

Those symptoms, when they start creeping back in and your remission is over, are a reminder that you were given a chance, and not to go back to your original way of life, to live for today, to believe in yourself and what you want to do. To reach for what you want. Surround yourself with the beauty that is friendship, the wonder that is love, and the contentment that comes with peace and compassion.

Make no mistake, I have lived well. I have traveled to more places and done more things than most people. I have selfishly spent on myself and generously helped others. I know how to flip a house to make money, landscape a home from dirt, and build a large piece of unassembled furniture. I can crochet, complete a crossword, pen and ink documents in Chancery Cursive, Early Uncials, and old English, and paint any room in a house.

I have been a season symphony ticket holder, seen Miles Davis play twice and been in the front row for many Rock and Country concerts and had as much fun at each as I did sitting in the nosebleed seats. I've been to major sporting events and enjoyed luxury suites. I have partied in limos and I have been to Vegas more times than a person should go. I have watched close friends get thrown by a bull, and I have danced until dawn, on several occasions.

I know the feeling of loving a child and having them love you. I know what it feels like to love unconditionally and to have that love returned by another human being, and I know the heartache of a lost young love and the pain of betrayal as I learned of a lover's infidelity.

I have had a friend brutally murdered and lost loved ones to accidental deaths and illnesses. I saw all four of my grandparents grow into old age gracefully and suffer with what ageing brings. I know what it is like to grow up in sibling rivalry and, as age and wisdom sets in, the joy that comes from rediscovering your sister's love and friendship.

I know what it feels like to have both parents love me, and for them to be there for me, to pick up the pieces without judgment.

I've learned how to walk away from painful, destructive, and hurtful relationship of all kinds, never to return, and the wonderment of being able to say "we've been friends for twenty years."

I have been lucky enough to have several people know me enough to call me their best friend. And to have been asked to be a godparent five times to the most amazing children.

I have written music and lyrics, blogs and poetry. I have laughed, cried, been scared and nervous. I have felt nothing and everything.

I have learned and grown from all these experiences that I was lucky enough to be a part of.

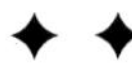

When given the opportunity to face your own mortality, things like this go through your head daily. The sun looks brighter, the flowers more colorful, and the stuff that once bothered you falls into nothingness.

My own mortality also made me want to shout louder than I ever had, to end the needless suffering of the people who are on chemotherapy drugs. To be the one to stand up and say loudly...

THIS SUCKS HELP US PLEASE.

Every one of us who suffers from these abominable, horrific, never-ending side-effects...

Literally... Until Death

Be Well~
Kim Henderly

I WOULD LIKE TO ACKNOWLEDGE AND THANK

My Other (Chris Henderly) - For being there when I didn't want to go forward. When it hurt too much. When I was too sick to move. For making me laugh when I wanted to cry. For loving me and holding my hand through the absolute worst of it all. You changed my life and my outlook. You made me a better person, and I can never thank you or love you enough for that. It proves that when you find your *other half* you can do anything.

The Little One (Hunter Henderly) - For saying the words that made me want to fight: "you can't leave me here." For sticking it out when you didn't have to. For smiling on the bad days. For making sure I ate and that I was warm. For forcing me to be strong and knowing that I can do this. You are a remarkable young man.

Bob & Pat Allegrina - For being there even when you are fighting your own battle. For all the years, all the trips, all the goodies. For the conversations and discussions. For the advice and the opinions. I couldn't have ordered better parents.

Sue and Ken Vaughn (Chris's Parent's) - For carting me to all my doctor's appointments, taking care of the little ones, helping us so that we may live comfortable and with less worry even on the worst of days. For being there for us always.

Michaelene & Ken Palyu - For bringing me treats and fixing our house. For giving up your weekends to work tirelessly to help us... over and over again.

Jennifer Perry - For all the hard-work you put in to help support me spiritually. Your gift of the soul and spirit is a blessing beyond words. Thank you for understanding that side of me.

Paula Lynch - For always being just a text away and helping in any little way that was asked of you and never once complaining about it. For your optimism in all this and the belief in its power is magical.

Charlotte Hobbs - My BFF, my other pea in the pod. For answering and looking up every question. For listening to me drone on and on about the same subject for years. For sharing the laughter and the pain. For never forgetting about me and what I like. For buying me treats, making me food and, most of all- sharing your family with me.

Sean P. Hobbs - For understanding your wife and mine's crazy friendship. For the advice and the incredible amount of your own personal time you spent on this project with me. For believing in all of this and standing shoulder to shoulder with me when others saw a different path. For knowing that I needed to yell this loudly.

Danielle & Brian Webb - For all your support, advice and assistance. For spending your vacation days taking care of me. Your unconditional friendship and laughter is so important to Chris and Me.

Mike and Jenn Balcom - For the laughter and the booze. For the music and the booze. For the friendship and the booze. For helping with all the shameless self-promotion. For the B-movies and the great times. For the emails, IMs, and texts. For understanding. I have loved every minute.

Bob Novosel - For knowing me enough to be the one who had to call and for never stopping. Your love and friendship over these past decades is everything to me. Your guidance and understanding has helped me be powerful and re-evaluate, even when I didn't want to. You are truly my brother.

Teri Selix - For sharing all your knowledge and experience. Your hard work, passion and fight is an inspiration.

Michelle Phillips-Baker – For caring and planning. For donating and helping. For being there and participating. You are an incredible woman.

Nathan Perry, Gavin Perry, Eddie Lynch V-For being my rays of sunshine. Your smiling faces, pure love and kindness make me smile every day.

Brooke Webb, Colin Hobbs, Ben Balcom and Kimberly Caramanoff - For being happy to see me even when I was bald. For smiling and laughing, for sitting on my lap and holding my hand even when I was scary sick. You all make me so happy.

Linda Freitag – For the incredible amount of meals you provided. For checking in on me and always volunteering to help.

Keith Hazely – For 'pulling the trigger'. For working around my crazy schedule and always being there to help me at every turn. You are an exceptional boss. Thank you for believing in me.

Nancy Hazely – For being an amazing woman. For not just being a run of the mill owner but an exceptional CEO with a grander vision for her company and team. For being a friend and a confidant. For letting me be my work-a-holic self and helping me cope with the boundaries this illness puts on a person with that type of personality. I am thankful every day that you were brought into my life.

Alison and Rich Donahee – For being the supportive friends that anyone would love to have in their life. For wanting me even when I'm sick to be part of your day. I cherish our friendship.

Kaitlin Moore and Patti Rose Lynch – You are the power I see in the women of the next generation. Carry forward... be strong, be brave and spread the word.

Joey Lynch, Eddie and Allisa Lynch – As I watched you grow into the wonderful adults you are... Hold tight that which is family. As you age you will need them more than ever.

Karen and Ken Stock - For always remembering and supporting me in so many ways.

The Wrobel's, The Staniec's, The Buscemi's, The Schmits, The Cicala's, The Dobrzycki, The Manczyk's, The Ortolan's, The Postma's, The Park's, The Cole's, The Volmer's, The Wysocki's, The Pilot and United Road Family – For the words of encouragement. The support in my cause. For helping in a way that I can never repay. Your family's support is immeasurable.

Melanie LaCasper – For the prayers and support. For being my biggest cheerleader.

David Chambers, Michelle Blake, Haley Dempster, Megan Savage, Roger Caramanoff, Trisha Kulesza, Tonya Nyberg, Carlo Barone, Mary Nugent, Faye Johnson, Ben Gonek, – For touching my life in the most positive way.

"I love each and every one of you more than you will ever know."